# NATURAL WOMAN

# NATURAL WOMAN

Herbal Remedies for Radiant Health
at Every Age and Stage of Life

↠ ↠ ↠ ↞ ↞ ↞

## DR. LESLIE KORN

SHAMBHALA
Boulder
2020

Shambhala Publications, Inc.
4720 Walnut Street, Boulder, Colorado 80301
www.shambhala.com

9 8 7 6 5 4 3 2 1

First Edition
Printed in the United States of America

⊗ This edition is printed on acid-free paper that meets the
American National Standards Institute Z39.48 Standard.
♻ This book is printed on 30% postconsumer recycled paper.
For more information please visit www.shambhala.com.

Shambhala Publications is distributed worldwide by
Penguin Random House, Inc., and its subsidiaries.

Designed by Laura Shaw Design

LIBRARY OF CONGRESS CATALOGING-IN-PUBLICATION DATA

Names: Korn, Leslie E., author.
Title: Natural woman: herbal remedies for radiant health at every age and stage of life /
Leslie Korn, PhD, MPH.
Description: Boulder: Shambhala, 2020. | Includes bibliographical references and index.
Identifiers: LCCN 2019013501 | ISBN 9781611806717 (paperback)
Subjects: LCSH: Herbs—Therapeutic use—Popular works. | Health—Popular works.
Classification: LCC RM666.H33 K674 2020 | DDC 615.3/21—dc23
LC record available at https://lccn.loc.gov/2019013501

# �》 CONTENTS 《⇠

# ⇢ PREFACE ⇠

I grew up a third-generation urban dweller. Is it any wonder that at age ten, I had a vision of going to the jungle and being a doctor amidst a forest of leaves, barks, and vines? At the age of twenty, I realized my youthful vision when I ventured to the jungles of western Mexico where I first learned about the use of foods and plants for healing. I lived in a coastal jungle village where there were no conventional doctors, and I was fortunate enough to get sick with almost everything possible because it gave me a chance to learn about the numerous subtropical diseases —not to mention the accidents, bites, and many maladies no one could name— I encountered during my first few years there. I learned about using herbs for healing as much from trial and error as from the women of the village. In essence, I served as my own laboratory, and I came to believe that this is a valuable way to learn about your health.

When I returned home to Boston ten years later, my grandmother Esther, who had just entered her ninth decade, told me that I came from a long line of women hailing from Romania who used herbs and foods as medicine. She shared with me all manner of healing treasures about our foremothers I had never known before. Apparently, healing was in my blood.

I have now been working as a healer, a clinician, and a health educator for over forty years. One of the things I always remind my students is that we started healing each other thousands of years ago, way before universities and credentialing bodies said that we could, and we have also had wise elders to whom we could turn for advice and new knowledge. This book is designed to serve as a wise elder resource for you to consult time and again for trusted guidance. Yet remember, too, that there may be times when seeking the help of a licensed health professional or specialist will be necessary in treating serious, unremitting health concerns.

# ⇒ ACKNOWLEDGMENTS ⇐

I traveled from my hometown in Boston on my way to the jungle of Mexico for the first time in 1973. En route, I stopped in Berkeley, California, for a week. During that week I went daily to a small bookstore on Telegraph Avenue called Shambhala Books. As a twenty-year-old feminist Jewish Buddhist and aspiring writer I thought, "Oh, I hope Shambhala will publish one of my books someday." Thus, I was thrilled when forty-three years later, I was approached by Beth Frankl, an editor at Shambhala, who shared with me a vision for this book that you are about to read. The seed for this book began on that avenue in Berkeley and was nourished by the years I spent learning about herbal medicines in a little village in rural Mexico that became my home for over forty years. Without Beth's invitation to write this book, publishing with Shambhala would have remained a long-forgotten dream. I am ever grateful to Beth Frankl for being part of the full circle this book represents as one of my treasured dreams as a writer.

Plants grow in communities, rarely thriving alone, and such is the case with a book like this one, whose development and life force benefited from the savvy of herbalists who worked with me as research assistants and interns, most notably herbalist Naneh Israelyn and skilled ethnobotanist and clinical herbalist Juliet Totten. These knowledgeable women provided research and ideas for rituals and formulas that they shared generously and, as a result, they gave breadth and depth to my work. My assistant, Leslie Sindos, is the essence of organization; she managed with aplomb the madness of an extraordinary amount of data, which enabled me to achieve the goals of this book. I could not imagine a better, more capable assistant. Alma Fátima Mora cheerfully brought her lyrical design to the book's companion website. My husband, Rudolph Ryser, is always a steadfast supporter. He was a joyful companion in the kitchen and the garden, as we created, tested, and tasted many of the recipes in this book, and he was a willing editor, hand-holder, and an ever-patient poet during the marathon of writing and in the final rush to the finish. I am indebted to him for making my often clumsy phrasing sing a bit more on key, and I am gifted by his presence in my life.

# ⇥ INTRODUCTION ⇤

Plant medicines can reduce and eliminate physical and emotional distress symptoms, act as women's allies in health, and bring balance and nourishment to our daily lives. They can also provide alternatives to many pharmaceuticals.

This book offers a compendium of commonly used herbs whose efficacy is supported by both indigenous and biomedical research. It is designed to serve as a companion to women and their children throughout all stages of their lives. The herbal medicines presented are practical resources for preventing illness and restoring health after acute and chronic illness. Many of these plants can be found in the backyard or on a local walk, but if you don't live near a particular plant or have time to pick your herbs at their most potent, you can purchase them at a special herbal apothecary or online. Once collected, you can store them in an herbal medicine cabinet or a first aid kit. Some special and unusual herbs and preparations, including herbs from Mexico, India, and the Mediterranean, may be new to you.

As you go through this book, you may find that you have an affinity for certain plants and feel drawn to them, and you may be repelled by others. As you discover these herbal medicines, you may use some of them over and over for a while and then suddenly find new ones as you continue to explore or have new needs. Using herbal medicines and integrating them into your life is an organic process.

In addition to information on herbs and their medicinal properties, I have included special instructions for using them in steams, poultices, and plasters relevant to women's health, along with explorations into women's biological rhythms and our entrainment to environmental rhythms, as they are central to our well-being. I also share stories about the role herbs have played in my own personal and professional life and healing.

## HOW TO USE THIS BOOK

There are many ways to get the answers you are seeking about using herbal medicines for your health. To help you do so, I have divided this book into chapters that allow you to search for information by action, herb name, health concern, or ritual. Chapter 1 provides a general introduction to herbs, including an explanation of how they heal, possible side effects, and the benefits of using the whole plant rather than just the active ingredient. It also provides a list of herb categories and the most important herbs in each. For example, if you are seeking to address stress, then you will want to understand "adaptogens" and know which herbs fall into that category.

Chapter 2 provides the basics of getting started. Included are ideas for acquiring herbs, along with ways to prepare them as medicines and the tools needed to do so. In chapter 3, you will learn how to create your own herbal medicine cabinet and first aid kit and the best herbs to include in each. Chapter 4 provides an alphabetical list of many important herbs and their benefits to our health. It's a good place to look up general information on an herb you are curious about. Chapter 5 provides delicious medicinal recipes for using herbs and spices daily for cooking, and chapter 6 is devoted to "spirit plants" and explores the use of entheogens and plants that alter states of consciousness and improve our mood and cognition. If you have a specific health concern, for example anxiety, insomnia, or polycystic ovary syndrome (PCOS), or you want to address menopausal symptoms, then you may look directly for the health topic or life stage issue in chapter 7 to see which herbs would be most helpful for your particular issue. I am especially excited to share ideas in chapter 8 for integrating herbs and ceremonial foods into rituals designed to celebrate and honor many of the major events we experience during our lives.

## SCIENTIFIC NAMES OF PLANTS

You will notice each plant also has a Latin name. These are called Latin binomials, the scientific names for each herb. While they might seem complicated, they are essential for knowing how to use herbs, especially as food or medicine, because using the wrong plant could be potentially dangerous.

Common names for plants vary geographically and culturally and can often refer to more than one plant. I see this when I travel from village to village in my work in Mexico, often finding many different plants called by the same name. No matter what language you speak, what region you call home, or which local plant names you have been taught, Latin binomials are universal, and therefore can reliably be used to correctly identify plants the world over.

One example of a common name referring to more than one species of plant is the case of chamomile. There are several species that are used medicinally, such as *Matricaria chamomilla* (German chamomile) or *Chamaemelum nobile* (Roman chamomile). These are both called chamomile, but they are two distinctly different species with different phytochemical properties. Another example is the common name plantain, which is used to describe a type of banana (*Musa*) as well as an herb (*Plantago major*).

Latin binomials are a map to each plant containing enough information to share a common language with anyone, anywhere. To break down the binomial let's explore the names for chamomile.

### MATRICARIA CHAMOMILLA (L.)

*Matricaria* refers to the genus, a taxonomic category that identifies a plant within a family. It is first in the name and always italicized and capitalized. *Chamomilla* is then the name of the specific species within the genus *Matricaria*. Species is always the second name in the binomial, not capitalized but italicized. The (L.) refers to Linnaeus, the name of the scientist who identified and categorized the species. The scientists' names are included in most academic texts but are often dropped in casual use of Latin binomials. In this text, I've opted not to use them. Latin binomials often change over time because taxonomists redefine the boundaries of what differentiates one species from another. Thus, crosschecking the scientific name of a plant you are interested in using by using multiple resources, old and new, can usually clarify the most current name.

## A WORD ABOUT BIOLOGY VS. GENDER

In this book I refer to a variety of herbs that address women's health challenges and stages of life. In many cases, I address health challenges that occur in the biologically female body, and in these instances, I am not referring to gender. Biologically, there is enormous diversity in hormone levels among all women, and while hormones do not define the person, they become salient when we are discussing the effects of herbs on hormones in our bodies. Women face many social, emotional, and cognitive challenges, as well as biological hurdles that may not align with their gender identity. I address this to the best of my ability and provide resources for topics that are beyond my expertise. Herbs play an important role in the lives of all women, and my hope is that this book explores this sacred connection between herbs and women in all their beautiful forms.

# NATURAL
# WOMAN

## ⇸⇸ 1 ⇷⇷

# HOW HERBS HEAL

Herbs are our first medicines. They are gifts from nature that grow out of the earth, nourished by the sun and the moon, the rain and the snow, to feed and heal us, nurturing our body, mind, and spirit. They remind us of our nature and enable us to live as women, naturally. So how do nature's herbs become medicines that heal us?

The word "medicine" is derived from the Sanskrit root word *mā*, meaning "measure" or "balance." Herbal medicines restore balance. They have specific, powerful compounds that function on many levels, causing physical or emotional responses in our body, mind, and spirit. So while their compounds or "active substances" can alter our physical bodies, they can also effect change energetically by bringing their spiritual vitalities to our electromagnetic energy fields. Some plants, like those I discuss in chapter 6, have psychoactive effects that cause changes in brain function that result in altered perception, mood, consciousness, cognition, or behavior. These plants are our allies as we discover new personal insights, enhance our connection to ourselves, others, and the cosmos, and possibly affirm our purpose and place in the world. They may also help to ease our fears as we prepare to leave our bodies to this earth.

While we may be tempted to apply only the science of biomedicine and say herbs work in support of our health because of a chemical or substance, we must do so with caution since these plant gifts come as a whole package. They work to combine all the elements necessary to provide balance, yes, but also to provide buffers to the potent active substances, which on their own can cause side effects.

Many of our well-known commercial pharmaceuticals are derived from herbal medicines. Researchers usually identify an active substance—what they consider the most important and useful part of the plant—and then extract it, concentrate it, and increase its potency to obtain a result. While this often works, it also can lead to other unexpected effects. When the compound is removed from the active parts of the whole plant that nature provided, it is also separated from all the other constituents that contribute to balance. For example, aspirin (acetylsalicylic acid) is derived from plants that belong to the genus *Spiraea*, which are rich in the analgesic (pain-killer) salicylic acid. Indigenous peoples have used many such plants both internally and externally for millennia. White willow bark (*Salix alba*) is one example. While aspirin is a powerful medicine, used to lessen pain, reduce fever, and thin the blood, it can have dangerous side effects, such as uncontrolled bleeding. It is also important to note that some people have what is called a "salicylate intolerance," and exposure to salicylates can cause asthma and hives.

Sugarcane (*Saccharum officinarum*) is another example of how extracting the powerful substance from the whole plant can lead to illness. When chewed as a food or herbal remedy or taken as freshly extracted juice, the sweet liquor is rich in micronutrients (iron, copper, manganese, zinc, molybdenum, and boron), minerals, trace amounts of B vitamins, and anti-inflammatory phenols. It is also used in India to treat jaundice and kidney diseases. For thousands of years, sugar was extracted from the grass and used like a spice—in small amounts—and it was very expensive. However, when sugar became commercially processed in large quantities as a granular sweetener and easily affordable, it brought new diseases like type 2 diabetes and heart disease.

Another example of the challenges of extracting compounds from whole plants is the coca leaf (*Erythroxylum coca*). Coca is rich in calcium, vitamins, and alkaloids and functions as a mild stimulant. Indigenous Quechua people chew coca leaves to prevent altitude sickness and also as an analgesic. When chewed in leaf form, coca is nonaddictive. It is only when the powerful alkaloids are extracted and concentrated in a powder form called "cocaine" and used separately from the whole plant that brain neurons are trampled, and addiction occurs.

Thus it is safe to say that while modern science has identified active substances for medicinal purposes, these substances do not always function well on their own; they exist as part of the complex intelligence of a whole plant. The task of healing ourselves and allowing the plant world to flourish is to decondition ourselves from treating the symptom alone with a chemical from a plant. Instead, we must seek to help our whole being with the whole plant and restore the capacity for balance and vitality.

That said, however, there are times when we need a powerful, directed, reliable response, for example an analgesic, antidepressant, or anxiolytic (an anxiety inhibitor). We want to ensure a rapid and sustained response based on principles of active substance, cofactors, synergists, measures, and ratios, long understood and studied by herbal scientists and pharmacists. In this book we explore how shaman and scientist alike apply herbal medicine.

## HERB, NUTRIENT, AND DRUG INTERACTIONS: CONTRAINDICATIONS AND SIDE EFFECTS

Every herb has the potential to cause side effects or to be contraindicated. Most contraindications in this book apply to pregnancy and breastfeeding. Some may apply to children or elders or are caused by interactions with pharmaceutical medicines. Herbs can enhance the actions of other medicines, or they can cause them to be excreted more quickly via the liver detoxification process. Some individuals may react differently than others because of genetics, biochemical sensitivities, or intolerances. Side effects can occur as a result of internal or topical application, inhalation leading to an allergic reaction, and contact dermatitis.

If you are currently taking medicines or high-dose nutritional supplements, it is essential to look up the herb you wish to use for any contraindications, its potential effects, and its interactions with the medicines or nutritional supplements you use. There are several online databases noted in the "Resources" section that allow you to identify interactions between herbs, nutritional supplements, or pharmaceutical drugs (prescription or over-the-counter) you are taking. However, consider that sometimes online databases offer contradictory information, requiring that we dig into the roots of knowledge, understand that the way research is carried out can lead to very different conclusions, and return to traditional empirical experience to help us navigate the confusion. For example ginseng root (*Panax ginseng*) extracts have exhibited inhibitory effects on human cancer cells, including breast cancer cells, in clinical research. Yet there remains conflicting evidence about whether ginseng possesses estrogenic activity that *proliferates* estrogen-dependent cancer cells. The seemingly contradictory data may be the result of different methods (water or alcohol) used in producing ginseng extracts. These challenges remind us to work with an herbalist or professional when making decisions about herbal protocols for cancer treatment. I have also found that some databases may be overly cautious in their warnings, especially about herbal interactions or use of herbs pre- and post-surgery. All of this points to the need to identify reliable support with an herbal specialist when determining your next steps.

## DEFINITIONS OF HERBAL ACTIONS AND SELECTED EXAMPLES

Herbs can be categorized according to how they act on our body and mind. These categories are listed here, along with examples of some of the most important herbs in each. Throughout the book I may refer to an herb in terms of one of these categories, so you may want to refer back to this list as you go along.

### ADAPTOGEN

Adaptogen plants help one adapt to stress by restoring the capacity to cope and respond. Along with their active extracts, they support adrenal function, build endurance, and reduce fatigue. By supporting adrenal function, they support immune function and resistance. They also help to utilize oxygen and increase cellular "breathing." Common adaptogenic herbs include ashwagandha (*Withania somnifera*), eleuthero (*Eleutherococcus senticosus*), also known as Siberian ginseng, and Korean ginseng (*Panax ginseng*).

### ALTERATIVE

Alterative herbs restore the body back to health after chronic or acute illness. They are nourishing, have a gentle effect on the body, and can be especially useful in cases of chronic inflammation and autoimmunity. Common alterative herbs include burdock root (*Arctium lappa*), cleavers (*Galium aparine*), garlic (*Allium sativum*), and plantain (*Plantago major*).

### ANODYNE/ANALGESIC

Anodyne or analgesic herbs are used topically or internally and work by decreasing the sensitivity of the nervous system to pain, thereby producing an analgesic effect. Common analgesic herbs include arnica (*Arnica montana*)—topical use only—corydalis (*Corydalis yanhusuo* and/or *Corydalis cava*), American skullcap (*Scutellaria lateriflora*), and white willow bark.

### ANTHELMINTIC

Anthelmintic herbs eliminate internal worms (helminths) from the digestive tract by either killing the worms (vermicide) or causing them to be eliminated (vermifuge), without causing significant damage to the host. Common varieties include hyssop (*Hyssopus officinalis*), tansy (*Tanacetum vulgare*), and wormwood (*Artemisia absinthium*).

### ANTICATARRHAL

Anticatarrhal herbs can clear excess mucus, and they tend to be used for upper respiratory ailments such as common colds or sinus infections. Common types include eyebright (*Euphrasia*), marshmallow (*Althaea officinalis*), mullein (*Verbascum thapsus*), goldenseal (*Hydrastis canadensis*), thyme (*Thymus vulgaris*), and yarrow (*Achillea millefolium*).

### ANTIDEPRESSIVE

Antidepressive herbs alleviate depression and improve mood and cognition. Common varieties include lemon balm (*Melissa officinalis*), oats (*Avena sativa*), pulsatilla (*Anemone pulsatilla*), saffron (*Crocus sativus*), and St. John's wort (*Hypericum perforatum*).

### ANTIDIPSOTROPIC

Antidipsotropic herbs reduce or help to prevent alcohol abuse. Common types include oats and kudzu (*Pueraria montana* var. *lobata*).

### ANTIEMETIC

Antiemetic herbs are used to relieve or halt vomiting and nausea. They can be used in cases of motion sickness or for nausea symptoms related to chemotherapy. Common antiemetic herbs include cannabis (*Cannabis sativa*), chamomile (*Matricaria chamomilla* and/or *Chamaemelum nobile*), ginger (*Zingiber officinale*), and peppermint (*Mentha piperita*).

### ANTIFUNGAL

Antifungal herbs destroy or inhibit fungal growth. Common varieties include garlic, olive leaf (*Olea europaea*), and tea tree (*Melaleuca alternifolia*).

### ANTIHEMORRHAGIC
Antihemorrhagic herbs are used to stop internal bleeding. They are generally drying herbs that encourage blood clotting. Common varieties include alfalfa (*Medicago sativa*), dong quai (*Angelica sinensis*), and yarrow.

### ANTI-INFLAMMATORY
Anti-inflammatory herbs regulate the inflammatory response in the body and reduce pain, heat, and other symptoms of inflammation. Common types include boswellia (*Boswellia serrata*), turmeric (*Curcuma longa*), and white willow bark.

### ANTILITHIC
Antilithic herbs dissolve or remove stones in the urinary system and can also prevent the stone from forming. Common varieties include horse gram (*Macrotyloma uniflorum*), hydrangea root (*Hydrangea arborescens*), and stonebreaker (*Phyllanthus niruri*).

### ANTIMICROBIAL
Antimicrobial herbs kill or inhibit the growth of microorganisms and can be taken for infections caused by bacteria, fungi, viruses, or parasites. Common varieties include garlic, oregano (*Origanum vulgare*), and Oregon grape root (*Berberis aquifolium*).

### ANTIPARASITIC
Antiparasitic herbs kill and expel parasites in the system. Common types include black walnut (*Juglans nigra*), goldenseal, papaya leaf and seeds (*Carica papaya*), and sweet Annie (*Artemisia annua*).

### ANTIPYRETIC/FEBRIFUGE
Antipyretic herbs prevent and reduce fevers. Common varieties include gotu kola (*Centella asiatica*), holy basil/tulsi (*Ocimum tenuiflorum*), and white willow bark.

### ANTISPASMODIC
Antispasmodic herbs ease and reduce muscle spasms and are used to relax muscles and organs that are tense and contracting. Common varieties include chamomile, hops, lobelia, myrrh gum, passionflower, American skullcap (*Scutellaria lateriflora*), and skunk cabbage (*Symplocarpus foetidus*).

## APERIENT

Often bitter in taste, aperient herbs stimulate bile and serve as mild laxatives that relieve constipation without stimulating peristalsis directly. Common types include burdock root, chamomile, and dandelion root (*Taraxacum campylodes*).

## APHRODISIAC

Aphrodisiac herbs enhance the capacity for sexual arousal. Common varieties include chocolate (*Theobroma cacao*), cordyceps (*Cordyceps*), damiana (*Turnera diffusa*), maca (*Lepidium meyenii*), and yohimbe (*Pausinystalia johimbe*).

## AROMATIC

Aromatic herbs, fragrant and rich in essential oils, stimulate the appetite by promoting the secretion of gastric juices. Common types include lavender (*Lavandula*), peppermint, rosemary (*Rosmarinus officinalis*), and sage (*Salvia officinalis*).

## ASTRINGENT

Astringent herbs help to dry excess moisture/secretions in the body. They tend to cause contractions in organ and muscle tissue and are typically high in tannins. Common astringent herbs include bearberry (*Arctostaphylos uva-ursi*), black tea (*Camellia sinensis*), oak (*Quercus*), and raspberry leaf (*Rubus idaeus*).

## BITTER

Bitter herbs stimulate digestion and appetite. They are tonifying to the liver and kidneys and promote the secretion of gastric juices. Common bitter herbs include dandelion greens and roots and gentian root (*Gentiana lutea*).

## CARDIOTONIC

Cardiotonic herbs strengthen the heart and circulatory system. Common varieties include hawthorn (*Crataegus*) and motherwort (*Leonurus cardiaca*).

## CARMINATIVE

Carminative herbs move gas and food through the bowels and reduce bloating and indigestion. Common types include anise seed (*Pimpinella anisum*), cardamom pod (*Elettaria cardamomum*), and fennel seed (*Foeniculum vulgare*).

## CHOLAGOGUE

Cholagogue herbs are often bitter and stimulate the secretion of bile. They are cleansing herbs that aid fat digestion and tonify the liver. Common cholagogue herbs include artichoke (*Cynara scolymus*), dandelion root, and gentian root.

## CHOLERETIC

Choleretic herbs increase bile secretions and are detoxifying with a gentle laxative effect. Common types include dandelion root, Oregon grape root, and turmeric.

## DEMULCENT

Demulcent herbs soothe the inflammation of dry, irritated tissue in respiratory conditions and ease the discomfort of urinary tract infections (UTIs). Common varieties include corn silk (*Zea mays*), marshmallow, and slippery elm bark (*Ulmus rubra*)

## DEPURATIVE

Depurative herbs detoxify the body by stimulating the natural cleansing abilities of the kidney and liver and purifying the blood. Common types include burdock root, cleavers, and dandelion leaf and root.

## DIAPHORETIC

Diaphoretic herbs promote sweating and are used to lower fevers. Common varieties include buchu (*Agathosma betulina*), burdock root, catnip (*Nepeta cataria*), and yarrow.

## DIURETIC

Diuretic herbs increase urination, remove excess water from the body, and flush out toxins. Common types include celery (*Apium graveolens*), dandelion leaf, goldenrod (*Solidago*), lovage (*Levisticum officinale*), and parsley (*Petroselinum crispum*).

## EMETIC

Emetic herbs are purgative and induce vomiting. They are appropriate for immediately expunging the contents of the stomach from poisoning. Common emetic herbs include blessed thistle (*Centaurea benedicta*), ipecac (*Carapichea ipecacuanha*), and lobelia (*Lobelia inflata*).

## EMMENAGOGUE

Emmenagogue herbs stimulate menstruation and increase blood to the pelvis and uterus. Common types include motherwort, rue (*Ruta graveolens*), and zoapatle (*Montanoa tomentosa*).

## EMOLLIENT

Emollient herbs are used as a topical treatment for dry, irritated skin. Common varieties include comfrey (*Symphytum officinale*), slippery elm bark, and spinach (*Spinacia oleracea*).

## EXPECTORANT

Expectorant herbs work by loosening bronchial secretions and mucus and easing congestion. They are usually classified by their mode of action, as either being stimulating or relaxing. Common expectorant herbs include the stimulating varieties such as elecampane (*Inula helenium*), ipecac, and mistletoe (*Viscum album*) and the relaxing varieties such as leek (*Allium ampeloprasum*), marshmallow, goldenseal, and thyme.

## GALACTAGOGUE

Galactagogue herbs stimulate the production of breast milk in nursing mothers. Common varieties include breadnut (*Brosimum alicastrum*), fennel seed, fenugreek seed (*Trigonella foenum-graecum*), and shatavari (*Asparagus racemosus*).

## HEPATIC

Hepatic herbs are liver tonics that work by strengthening and tonifying the liver tissue and by increasing bile production. Common types include beet root and greens (*Beta vulgaris*), milk thistle (*Silybum marianum*), and schisandra (*Schisandra chinensis*).

## HORMONE MODULATING

Hormone modulating herbs bring homeostasis to hormonal imbalance. They usually contain constituents of similar structure to certain hormones produced by the human body and so bind to corresponding hormone receptor sites, with slight agonistic effect. Common hormone modulating herbs include chasteberries (*Vitex agnus-castus*) and wild yam (*Dioscorea villosa*).

## HYPNOTIC

Hypnotic herbs sedate, relax, and help one sleep. While similar in action to sedatives, hypnotics are often more powerful in nature. Common hypnotic herbs include Jamaican dogwood (*Piscidia piscipula*) and kava kava, or simply kava (*Piper methysticum*).

## HYPOGLYCEMIC

Hypoglycemic herbs lower and regulate raised blood sugar levels. Common varieties include bitter melon (*Momordica charantia*), cinnamon (*Cinnamomum verum*), and damiana.

## HYPOTENSIVE

Hypotensive herbs lower and regulate blood pressure. Common types include garlic, hawthorn, and stinging nettle (*Urtica dioica*).

## IMMUNOMODULATING/IMMUNOSTIMULATING

Immunomodulating herbs affect immune responsiveness; immunostimulating herbs are nonspecific and used for acute conditions. These herbs are often classified as either deeply activating or surface activating/immune boosting. Common immunomodulating herbs include reishi (*Ganoderma*) and schisandra; common immunostimulating herbs include echinacea (*Echinacea purpurea*) and myrrh (*Commiphora myrrha*).

## LAXATIVE

Laxative herbs relieve constipation by causing bowel movements. Laxatives are often classified by their different modes of action. Aperients (see page 6) are bulking laxatives that draw water into the colon, in turn softening and adding bulk to the stool. Stimulating laxatives, which contain constituents that cause contractions within the muscle of the digestive tract, encourage movement of stool. Common laxative herbs include bulking varieties such as flaxseed (*Linum usitatissimum*) and psyllium husk (*Plantago indica*), and stimulating varieties include cascara sagrada (*Frangula purshiana*), rhubarb (*Rheum rhabarbarum*), and senna (*Senna alata*).

CAUTION: Stimulating laxatives can cause discomfort in the abdominal region and should not be used long term.

## NERVINE

Nervines are defined by their action on the nervous system: they can tonify, relax, or stimulate. Nervine tonics, also called trophorestoratives, strengthen the whole system, while relaxing herbs aid sleep, reduce pain, or soften digestive distress. Stimulants may lift mood and reduce fatigue. Common nervine herbs include nervine tonics such as oat, bacopa (*Bacopa monnieri*), and passionflower (*Passiflora edulis*), nervine relaxants such as kava, lavender, and St. John's wort, and nervine stimulants such as coffee (*Coffea arabica*), ginseng, and peppermint.

## PARTURIENT

Parturient herbs induce and promote labor and/or are beneficial during pregnancy. Common varieties include partridge berry (*Mitchella repens*) and red raspberry (*Rubus idaeus*). **NOTE:** There is now consensus among herbalists to stop recommending blue cohosh during all phases of pregnancy, though it is still sometimes used in labor by midwives. This is further discussed in chapter 4.

## RUBEFACIENT

Rubefacient herbs increase circulation to a localized area when applied topically. They are used for painful musculoskeletal conditions, like fibromyalgia, or to draw blood to the surface, and they tend to cause redness and heat. Common rubefacient herbs include cayenne (*Capsicum annuum*), horseradish (*Armoracia rusticana*), mustard (*Brassica juncea, Brassica nigra* and/or *Sinapis alba*), and stinging nettle.

## SEDATIVE

Sedatives are nervine herbs that promote sleep and relaxation. Common types include California poppy (*Eschscholzia californica*), hops (*Humulus lupulus*), and valerian (*Valeriana officinalis*).

## SPASMOLYTIC. *See* "Antispasmodic."

## STIMULANT

Stimulant herbs increase awareness, alertness, and memory and energize and boost mood. Common types include ginger, ginkgo (*Ginkgo biloba*), gotu kola, and rosemary.

## STYPTIC

Styptic herbs are used to stop external bleeding. Common varieties include calendula (*Calendula officinalis*), cayenne pepper, and yarrow.

## THYMOLEPTIC. *See* "Antidepressive."

## TONIC

*Tonic* is a broadly applied term that refers to herbal agents that work in a variety of ways to strengthen and tone the body. Tonics are often specific to a particular organ or system, e.g., a uterine tonic or kidney tonic. Common tonic herbs include ginger, gotu kola, holy basil/tulsi, oats, and American skullcap.

### TROPHORESTORATIVE

Trophorestorative herbs strengthen and restore the vitality of tissue, and most have an affinity for one particular organ or system. Common varieties include oats and American skullcap for the nervous system, milk thistle for the liver, licorice (*Glycyrrhiza glabra*) for the endocrine system, and mullein for the respiratory system).

### UTERINE ASTRINGENT

Uterine astringents are used to tonify the uterus and reduce excessive blood loss in menstruation. Common varieties include lady's mantle (*Alchemilla xanthochlora*), red raspberry, and yarrow.

### UTERINE NERVINE

Uterine nervines (*see also* "Nervine") have an affinity for the uterus and surrounding reproductive organs. They nourish and support overall nervous sytem function. Some, like mugwort, are relaxing while others, like cramp bark, are antispasmodic. Common types include black cohosh root (*Actaea racemosa*) and American skullcap (*Scutellaria lateriflora*).

### VULNERARY

Vulnerary herbs are used to heal wounds, either external or internal. Common types include calendula, comfrey, and yarrow.

## CONCLUSION

Understanding the many ways herbs act on the body and mind provides us with options to use them daily for our optimal health, for both acute emergenices and to prevent and treat chronic illness. Herbs are classified by how they affect organ function and whole systems, like the endocrine or immune system. They may stimulate or relax us by increasing or decreasing the release of chemicals, and they work in myriad ways to bring about a desired effect. Some, like adaptogens, have general nonspecific effects that enhance our ability to cope with stress. Many herbs serve many functions at once, such as how hawthorn is often used as a cardiotonic, anthelmintic, and anxiolytic. Herbs certainly have chemicals that affect our health but as we use herbs, we are also mindful that nature has provided us with the whole plant for a reason; the combination of nutrients, chemistry, and life force that brings healing to us acts in concert to achieve balance, known as *mā*, the foundation for lasting health and well-being.

## ⇉ ⇉ 2 ⇇ ⇇

# PREPARING YOUR HERBAL MEDICINES

## TOOLS AND METHODS

T here is much to know about finding herbs and preparing them for prevention, healing, and culinary delights. In this chapter I provide you with suggestions on how to acquire your herbs, factors to consider when deciding on the best way to use them, and instructions and recipes for preparing them.

### ACQUIRING HERBS

Herbs can be purchased, harvested, or collected, and you'll need to choose the options that suit your locality and lifestyle. I love growing culinary herbs in my indoor and outdoor kitchen gardens. They are simple to cultivate, and there is nothing like picking some fresh rosemary for my roasted potatoes or a fresh chili off the vine to give some spice to my cognac damiana cocktail.

Turning your lawn into an herbal garden is another sustainable way to have a steady supply of herbs that will nourish you throughout the year. And, of course, many plants such as the valuable and vigorous dandelion and milk thistle pop up on their own every spring and summer. These herbal remedies arrive just in time for my liver spring-cleaning for which I make some of my own medicines in the form of teas, salves, extracts, and cordials (see my recipes in the "Spring Cleanse" section on pages 41–45).

I also purchase and store pharmaceutical-grade medicines that I want to have on hand. These are remedies that are made from herbs from other countries or that may involve a more complicated or time-consuming process for which I can't or do not want to devote time and energy.

If you live in an urban area, it is often easier to purchase herbs than to grow or collect your own. A day or weekend trip away, however, may allow you to wildcraft your own herbs. There are also many herbal schools and community-supported agricultural farms in close proximity to urban areas, so a trip to pick herbs could be just a short drive away. Or if you volunteer at a farm, a basketful of fresh herbs could be yours for the picking.

I enjoy the benefits of herbal wisdom and practices from all over the world, so I look to experts who engage in thoughtful, ethical herbal collection practices. For example, kava, a powerful root whose name is derived from the Polynesian word *awa*, meaning "bitter," is only available in the South Pacific. I'll often research the names of people collecting it and ask them if the kava has been thoughtfully harvested and in collaboration with the local indigenous peoples, and if it has been carefully prepared with attention to potency and safety. If I receive satisfactory answers to these questions, I can then decide if I want kava-based capsules, extract, or root to prepare as a tea for when I want to relax or am feeling anxious.

## SAFEGUARDING ENDANGERED PLANTS

Many herbs are on the verge of extinction due to overharvesting or the effects of climate change. Scientists are also discovering that the rising $CO_2$ in the atmosphere is changing the chemistry and nutritional value of plants we have relied on for centuries. As you explore ways to acquire your herbs, consider whether the herbs you wish to use are best collected in the wild, grown in the garden, or purchased from ethical sources. United Plant Savers is an organization involved in raising awareness about plants at risk and promoting actions to conserve them. This doesn't mean they cannot be used, just that we need to stay aware of how we access and use them so we can safeguard them for generations to come. The following plants have been identified as at risk:

American ginseng (*Panax quinquefolius*)

Bloodroot (*Sanguinaria canadensis*)

Black cohosh (*Actaea racemosa*)

Blue cohosh (*Caulophyllum thalictroides*)

Echinacea (*Echinacea*)

Eyebright (*Euphrasia*)

False unicorn root (*Chamaelirium luteum*)

Goldenseal (*Hydrastis canadensis*)

Lady's slipper orchid (*Cypripedium*)

Lomatium (*Lomatium dissectum*)

Osha root (*Ligusticum porter*)

Peyote (*Lophophora williamsii*)

## HARVEST AND USE INVASIVE PLANTS

When I lived in Olympia, the Department of Natural Resources "sheriff" knocked on my door one day and said, "You have milk thistle growing in your yard, and you need to remove it." I asked him why, since I was so proud of the beautiful thistles (they needed no help from me), and I was waiting to harvest their seeds to make liver medicine. I did not know that it was considered a noxious plant in the state of Washington and dangerous to cattle and other grazing animals. The sheriff was understanding of my intentions and agreed to let me wait the five more days I needed for a successful harvest.

Like milk thistle, many plants are considered noxious or invasive for a wide range of reasons, and yet they are also wonderful medicines. Some of these plants, such as kudzu, plantain, knotweed (*Polygonum*), blackberries (*Rubus allegheniensis*), English ivy (*Hedera helix*), and Scotch broom (*Cytisus scoparius*), are only considered invasive in certain areas of the country or the world because they may be nonnative, they affect farmers' crops, or are dangerous to livestock. Your local county weed board will have identified the plants growing in your area that have been classified as noxious or invasive. Explore where you may harvest these plants and then prepare them as medicines to your heart's content. Remember, many counties spray these plants under their mandatory removal programs (in contrast to less aggressive containment programs) and you will want to ensure that you collect unsprayed plants.

| ⇝ *22 Ways to Integrate Herbs into Your Life Right Now* ⇐ |
|---|

1. Eat fresh herbs.
2. Freeze fresh herbs in ice cubes and serve in your favorite beverage.
3. Sip herbal iced teas.
4. Add herbs to your morning smoothie.
5. Make pesto with different herbs.
6. Add herbs to your stocks, broths, and sauces.
7. Use spices when cooking.
8. Add ginger and cinnamon to your morning oats.
9. Add a pinch of ground cayenne pepper to your hot chocolate.
10. Buy tinctures or capsules.
11. Make a first aid kit.
12. Make a sleep pillow.
13. Make an herbal wreath for the holidays.
14. Go on an herb walk.
15. Interview a wise elder about their use of herbs.
16. Undertake a ritual using herbs.
17. Make herbal vinegars.
18. Infuse olive oil with herbs.
19. Create herbal cocktails and "mocktails."
20. Grow a kitchen garden inside and out.
21. Plant a chamomile lawn.
22. Make a salve and give it away as gifts during holidays

## PREPARATION

Herbs add flavor to our cuisine and are consequently closely tied to food preparation. How we prepare herbs depends on how we plan to use them. Whether we wish to dry them and store them for future use or prepare a fresh delight each day, our herbs are ready to support our health, excite our palate, boost our energy, or calm us for a good night's sleep. Herb quality can degrade when exposed to sunlight and UV rays and to protect herbal preparations you will note that I often suggest using amber glass covered jars or storing herbs in a dark cabinet. Now let's look more closely at methods for preparing our precious herbs.

When preparing to make herbal remedies I ask the following questions:

- What type of preparation does this herb need to enhance its efficacy? For example, is this herb best taken as a tea and if so, do I infuse the leaves or boil the roots for 20 minutes? Or should I make a pomade or soak in a bath and absorb the herb's qualities through my skin?

- How much time do I need to prepare my remedy? Is it an emergency and if so, do I need to find a preparation at a store or do I have time to make it at my leisure? If I make it and want to have it on hand for the future, how long will it last and under what conditions should I store it?

- Is the herbal remedy I need complex or simple to prepare? Do I have the time and know-how to do it?

- If I prepare this herbal remedy, can I make enough to last for a few days or weeks or is it better to make it fresh each time?

- Do I need to wait before I can use the remedy? For example, does it need to macerate for a month or more in order to be effective?

- How do I like to take herbs and what will enhance my adherence to my prevention or treatment plan? For example, if I don't like swallowing capsules, then I might prefer to take a liquid or add a powder to my smoothie.

- Are there family members or friends who will join me in making these preparations? Shall I organize an herbal medicine-making event?

- What tools do I need to make my remedies?

## EQUIPMENT

We don't need anything fancy to use herbs successfully; however, a few choice pieces of equipment will serve many purposes in the kitchen and get you off to a good start. For instance, if you are going to cook with herbs, a slow cooker and a blender or food processor are your best options. When making heated herbal oils, a double boiler helps, and if you are going to grind seeds, a *molcajete* (a Mexican mortar and pestle) and an electric grinder are next on your list. You can build your equipment piece by piece over time, or better yet, make up your perfect herbal medicine gift list so when family and friends ask you what you want for your birthday, you can tell them that you would appreciate a blender, slow cooker, dehydrator, diffuser, electric grinder, molcajete, muslin bags, stainless steel or glass pots (no aluminum please), strainers, amber glass jars, and cheesecloth.

## PREPARING YOUR HERBAL MEDICINES

The ways to incorporate herbs into your life are limitless. Among these delivery methods are teas, tinctures, extracts, glycerites, steams, soaks, rubs, salves, steams, smoke and vape baths and soaks, water infusions and decoctions, oils, syrups, elixirs, cordials, honeys, vinegars, oxymels, herbal-infused oils, pills, capsules, lozenges, and suppositories. In the next section I will walk with you in a garden of delights where you begin to sip, drink, soak, pucker, and insert a variety of herbs that will serve your health and well-being.

### BATH/SOAK

A soak is an herbal-infused bath that relieves distress, soothes painful musculoskeletal conditions, and alleviates skin issues. Foot soaks are helpful in cases where a bathtub is not available. Adding herbs to a basin of hot water makes a relaxing remedy for painful, tired feet. A simple way to prepare an herbal bath is to stuff a muslin bag with herbs and place it in the hot water.

→ *My Favorite Herbal Bath Soak* ←

After a long day I fill the tub with hot water and add a cup of Epsom salt (magnesium sulfate), which relaxes the muscles and the mind. I then add 5 to 10 drops of attar of rose oil and soak for 20 minutes. As the rose oil dissipates, I add 5 drops of lavender oil and I am ready for a deep sleep.

### CORDIAL/ELIXIR

Cordials are made with fresh plants, and elixirs are made with dried herbs. The word *cordial* refers to the heart. (Think of being cordial to someone.) Cordials are yummy medicinal beverages with about 30 to 50 percent alcohol by volume that combine medicinal plants with liquor and honey to warm the heart and relax the mind. They are best imbibed in the afternoon through late evening (though having a rough day might call for one in early afternoon). Using small amounts of cordials and elixirs is a good way to deliver herbal medicine to elders, and cordials are ideal for rituals celebrating love.

To make a cordial, you'll need an amber glass quart jar. Fill half the jar with a mixture of plants and ground seeds, and then fill the rest of the jar with your choice of alcohol. I use brandy, sherry, or a fine tequila. Make sure the herbs are completely covered and leave a little space at the top of the jar for the expansion of the plants. Tightly screw on the lid and label the the jar with the contents and date. Store in a cool, dark closet and steep the herbs for at least a month.

After a month, strain the liquid into a clean jar and add ¼ cup of raw honey, grade B maple syrup, or a touch of blackstrap molasses. Or get creative and add dried fruits for extra added sweetness. If you used brandy or sherry, the cordial will be naturally sweet, so you won't need to add as much sweetener. This cordial/elixir can be kept at room temperature for many years.

## » My Favorite Fennel Cordial «

A digestive cordial is the perfect way to start or end a meal. Digestion begins with relaxation. If we are not relaxed when we eat, the fiery digestive enzymes will not be released, and digestion will be difficult. This is why we can get heartburn when we are stressed. Sitting down for an herbal cordial before dinner sets the stage for relaxation and having one after dinner provides the digestive system with soothing and carminative herbs. The following combination of herbs is an Ayurvedic remedy, and it works beautifully as a cordial.

**MAKES 4 CUPS**

3 ounces fennel seed

2 ounces fenugreek seed

1 ounce licorice root

4 thumbs fresh ginger, cut into slices

16 ounces brandy

¼ cup raw local honey

Grind the fennel seed, fenugreek seed, and licorice root in an electric herb or coffee grinder and add the mixture to an amber glass quart jar. Then add the ginger slices. Pour over the brandy, screw the lid on the jar tightly, and let sit for 1 month in a dark corner, shaking gently a few times a week. Strain the liquid into a new jar and add the honey. Sip before or after a meal to aid digestion and prevent or reduce gas and discomfort.

## DECOCTION

A decoction is a method of extraction by heating plant material in water. This preparation is usually done for the woody parts of plants, like rhizomes, bark, twigs, berries, or mushrooms. In a small pot, put 1 ounce of herbs in 1 quart of water and simmer on low for 20 to 45 minutes. For a stronger brew and more potent medicine, simmer the liquid until it is reduced to a concentrate. Leaves, flowers, and herbs high in volatile oils, like valerian root or fennel, do not do well in decoctions, as simmering eradicates many of their important medicinal compounds.

## ELECTUARY

An electuary is made from powdered herbs and honey for topical or internal use. Honey is the most important *anupana* (vehicle of administration) in Ayurvedic medicine. It is also a *yogavahi* in Ayurveda, which means that it potentiates the herbs that are taken with it. To make an herbal-infused honey with dried herbs, cover the leaf or root with honey and let it sit on a windowsill or in a cupboard (not too hot) for 6 weeks. Powdered herbs are easier to use in this preparation, as you will not have to strain them afterward. If you use fresh herbs or flowers like roses, make sure that they dry thoroughly before adding them to the honey. If you choose to use unprocessed herbal material, pour it through a mesh strainer once the honey is finished infusing. Once the honey is ready, it may be added to desserts and salad dressings or, if you infused it with garlic, use it for cold and flu prevention.

### ⇻ The Uses of Honey ⇺

Honey is an important ingredient in herbal medicine. Honey is made by bees from the nectar of various local wildflowers, many of which are medicinal—for example, echinacea, dandelion, and valerian. The nectar from these plants contains the same medicinal actions of the plants themselves.

Honey is antibiotic, antiviral, and anti-inflammatory and can be used as an expectorant, laxative, and tonic. Because it is rich with minerals, vitamins, antioxidants, and natural enzymes, it can also be used to nourish the skin. When applied topically, honey allows the skin to retain moisture, making it an excellent remedy for healing dry skin and wounds. It also absorbs excess oil, which makes it useful in the treatment of acne. Honey is highly effective in coating the throat to soothe coughs and throat irritation and in stimulating salivation, which in turn thins mucus and acts as an expectorant. People with pollen allergies may benefit from eating the honey made in their neighborhood as an immunotherapy that provides exposure to small amounts of the substance that causes reactions in larger exposures and may reduce reactivity over time.

## FERMENTATION

Fermentation is used to preserve food, improve digestibility, and support the absorption of food. It breaks down plant materials to their more basic constituents and creates new compounds including enzymes, organic acids, and antioxidants.

Fermentation supports our gut, or "second brain," the garden of our body where our bacteria flourish to promote our digestion and cocreate mood chemicals for our first, or primary, brain. Our mood and focus are so dependent on a well-functioning gut and a lively garden of bacteria that these fermented products are now call "psychobiotics."

There are so many ways to ferment herbs, plants, fruits, and vegetables and if we study the world's cultures (pun intended!), we discover that every community ferments some food in order to stay healthy. Try this herbal tepache recipe for starters. It's a great way to put the skins and core of the pineapple to work after you eat the fruit. A tepache can be served as a fermented beverage or used as a base for other recipes like salad dressings, in which you can use it in place of vinegar.

### ⇉ *Pineapple Herbal Tepache* ⇇

**MAKES 2 CUPS**

Skin and core of one pineapple

2 cups filtered water

3 thumbs fresh ginger, unpeeled

7 thumbs fresh turmeric root or
    2 tablespoons dried powdered
    root, unpeeled

2 tablespoons raw local honey

1 tablespoon ground cayenne
    pepper

In a blender or food processor combine the pineapple skin, water, ginger, turmeric, honey, and cayenne and blend until mostly juiced, if a little pulpy. Chop the core of the pineapple and combine with the juiced ingredients in a large glass pitcher. Cover the mixture with a clean dishcloth secured with a rubber band to allow fermentation gases to be released. Allow the pitcher to rest on the counter at room temperature for 2 days. After 2 days, skim any accumulated foam off the top of the mixture, re-cover, and allow it to rest for another day (or two, if preferred) of fermentation. Finally, strain the mixture through a fine mesh sieve into a clean jar or pitcher, compost the solids, and enjoy your tepache!

## GLYCERITE

A glycerite is an herbal remedy that uses vegetable glycerin as the extraction medium for the herbal material. Glycerites tend to taste better and are more suitable than alcohol for children, or those with an alcohol intolerance. Glycerites have a shorter shelf life than alcohol tinctures, lasting up to 2 years. To make a glycerite, fill an amber glass quart jar halfway with chopped dried herbs. In a separate mixing bowl, make a mixture of 2 cups of 75% vegetable glycerin and 25% distilled water and then pour the mixture over the herbs, filling the jar to the top. Screw on the lid tightly. Soak the herbs for 4 to 6 weeks in a cool, dry place, shaking daily. When it's ready, strain the liquid into a clean jar, compost the solids, and label the glycerite with the date and contents.

## HERBAL CAPSULES

Herbal capsules are made by grinding herbs and then funneling the material in pre-purchased gelatin capsules. You can combine different herbs to create your own medicinal formula. This process is rather laborious but once done, you should have enough medicine to last for up to 6 months, especially if you store the capsules in an amber glass jar away from sunlight. Capsules are great for those who are not a fan of the taste of herbs. However, those who have difficulty swallowing capsules will obviously not benefit from this mode of therapy.

## HERBAL LINIMENT

Linaments are designed to be rubbed on the skin with vigor to reduce pain, stimulate circulation, or relieve aching joints. While often made with alcohol (and sometimes oil) I prefer alcohol-free witch hazel because you get the benefits of the soothing witch hazel, which is rich in tannins as well as the herb you are soaking. The elders in the jungle taught me how to make my first liniment by soaking a handful of *mota* (cannabis) in *raicilla* (local moonshine made from the stem of the agave) for a few weeks. The local *sobadores* then used it for massaging anyone who fell from a horse or out of a boat or hammock, adding a few drops under the tongue for good measure. Make this liniment jungle style: grab a handful of cannabis, add it to an amber glass jar, cover it with alcohol, cap tightly, and let it sit for 14 days until it's ready for use. No need to strain, just pour it onto sore muscles and rub. Make your liniments in advance and store them in the cupboard so you have them on hand for those late-night aches and pains.

## HERBAL OIL

Herbal oils are made using heat to infuse plant material in a high-quality oil. To prepare an herbal oil, cover plant material with olive, almond, or coconut oil, cap tightly, and let it sit in an amber glass jar for a few weeks on a warm, sunny windowsill or outside during the summer months to use solar energy to warm and blend the healing energies. Alternatively, make it quickly by heating the oil and herbs in a double boiler on a low simmer for 2 hours, then strain and bottle the oil. Herbal oils are perfect for adding to our daily diet or applying topically.

### ➤ *Topical Herbal-Infused Sunlight Oil* ←

Arnica simmered in almond oil makes an all-purpose skin tonic and bruise healer. There are two kinds of arnica: *Arnica montana* and *Arnica mexicana* (*Heterotheca inuloides*); both are anti-inflammatory and should be used only topically.

Make this oil and bottle it in 2-ounce amber glass bottles and give it for holiday gifts. People always need arnica oil and it's a staple of my first aid kit.

Fill a wide-mouthed amber glass quart jar ¾ full with dried arnica flowers and some arnica leaves. Make sure they are completely dry, so they don't develop mold. Cover the flowers with almond oil or virgin cold-pressed olive oil, leaving 3 inches at the top of the jar, and cover. Place in a warm, sunny location for 3 to 4 weeks and then strain the oil through cheesecloth, squeezing out all the oil from the plant material. Then bottle the liquid into small amber or green glass jars and store away from light. For a variation, add a few whole dried African bird peppers to the oil for some gentle heat.

## HERBAL PILLS

Herbal pills are powdered herbal material mixed with water and hand rolled into an ingestible tablet. You can buy herbs already in powdered form—or grind your own—and mix them with water until the consistency of the mixture is doughy. Some people suggest using a binding material, such as starch or natural gum, to keep the mixture from losing its consistency. However, if you immediately place the rolled pills into the freezer, they will keep until you need to take them. These pills are more suited to fibrous plant parts, such as roots or bark, than to leaves.

## HERBAL VINEGARS

Herbal vinegars are liquid extracts that use vinegar as the main solvent. They are excellent for children and for those who cannot consume alcohol. Vinegars can be consumed as a food or used in baths and are especially useful when you are fatigued or anxious. Herbal vinegars can be made by soaking the herbal material in vinegar—apple cider vinegar is one of the best to use—for 2 weeks in a dry, cool place, and later straining it until all the herbal material is gone. Herbal vinegars can be mixed into dressings, beverages, marinades, and other meals; however, for medicinal benefit, 1 to 2 tablespoons of the herbal vinegar 3 times a day is effective.

## » *My Favorite Vinegar Bath and Herbal Soak* «

I work with a lot of patients who experience anxiety, depression, and fatigue, and there is no better pick-me-up than an herbal bath or foot soak. Vinegar acidifies the body and counteracts the alkalinizing effect of the shallow breathing that goes with anxiety or even too much lettuce in the diet! For a simple vinegar bath, add 1 cup of white or apple cider vinegar to the water and soak for 20 minutes. Within 3 days your energy and mood will pick up and your breath will find its rhythm. I make my herbal bath soak in advance and keep it in the fridge for up to a week at a time.

In a large mixing bowl, add 4 tablespoons each of dried lavender and peppermint, and then pour in 1 quart of apple cider vinegar. Mix well and strain, and then store the liquid in a glass quart jar in the fridge until you need it. When you're ready for your soak, add 1 cup of the vinegar to a hot bath—the aroma of the peppermint will dissolve a headache and brighten your mood, and the lavender will soothe the stress away. You can do these baths any time of day but consider doing the vinegar bath early in the day and the herbal bath soak with Epsom salt (page 18) at night to aid sleep.

### INFUSION

An infusion is made when you let herbs soak in cold or hot water. Tea is a type of infusion (see page 28). Making a cold infusion requires soaking 1 ounce of herb in a quart of room temperature water for 8 hours and then straining. The same ratios apply to a hot infusion, but soaking can be accomplished in 4 hours or less. A quick tea infusion can be made in 15 minutes.

### LOZENGE

To make a lozenge, brew a strong herbal infusion or decoction. Among the best herbs to use for a sore throat lozenge will be slippery elm, elderberry, lemon zest, and ginger. Strain and add back into a saucepan and add honey to it. Heat it on high until it bubbles up around the pan, stirring constantly with a wooden spoon. Then lower the heat and let it thicken for another 10 minutes until almost all of the water is removed, then pour the liquid into candy molds. Once the lozenges have almost hardened, sprinkle more of the powdered herb on the molds and store in the fridge or freezer.

## → *Slippery Elm Lozenges* ←

Slippery elm is such a magical and versatile plant that is healing just from the smell of the earthen bark. Slippery elm bark makes the best lozenges for calming a cough because it soothes mucous membranes from the mouth to the esophagus, lungs, and colon. Slippery elm is also a nourishing food that native peoples of the northern climes traditionally use to supplement scarce food supplies, so sucking on lozenges when you're sick will speed healing even when you're not eating much. Old herbalist lore suggests that during preparation, you'll want to simmer the bark twice to bring out all the best qualities of the herb. Slippery elm lozenges are also available commercially.

### OIL PULLING
Oil pulling is an ancient Ayurvedic method of detoxification and balancing the microbiome in the mouth using cold-pressed sesame or coconut oil. Coconut oil is antibacterial and rich in lauric acid. It is made even more effective by adding a few drops of myrrh essential oil, which is antibacterial and antiviral, along with a few drops of cinnamon or mint essential oil as a mouth freshener. Brush your teeth first, then take 1 to 2 tablespoons of oil and swish it around in your mouth for 10 to 20 minutes. As you swish, allow it to travel around the mouth, so the oil and herbs can stimulate the salivary glands that allow for herbal absorption.

### OINTMENT
An ointment is a topical preparation made with an oil base that has medicinal herbs added for treatment. While I was in the jungle, I banged my bare toe on a rock during a rainstorm, and then while I was walking, the animal feces on the dirt path found my toe and within a day I had a full-blown staph infection. So I decided to test the antibiotic power of fresh topical garlic. It took 10 days of 3 daily applications of garlic ointment (see page 26), foot soaking, drying, and leg elevation but the infection finally cleared. If I had been able to see a physician, I might have been prescribed

a 10-day dose of antibiotics. Nature heals, but it often takes more work and more time than our modern pharmaceuticals (though in this case it was about the same). The key is to make informed decisions about all the options: what we actually need for ourselves and our families and what represents the safest approach at the time.

## → *Garlic Ointment* ←

This ointment can be used to treat a topical bacterial or fungal infection. Take 12 peeled cloves of fresh garlic and crush them in a molcajete or blend them in a blender. Then add ¼ cup of coconut oil. Garlic is a powerful antibiotic, and coconut oil is antibacterial and antifungal. Apply the ointment to the affected area 3 times a day and cover lightly with a new gauze bandage after each application. The key is to treat the infection with the antibacterial, while also giving the wound a chance to breathe during the day. Take 1 to 2 capsules of oregano oil, 3 times a day to support antibacterial action internally. Use for 10 days only.

CAUTION: If after 48 hours it appears the infection is getting worse (if the swelling and redness increases), then do not wait to seek medical help. Garlic will often work, but at times a pharmaceutical antibiotic will be necessary.

### OXYMEL

An oxymel is a mixture of acid, usually vinegar, and honey, which is often made to mask the taste of strong or nasty tasting herbs. The combination of honey and vinegar is also healing in itself during an illness that weakens the appetite. There are two methods for making one: the first uses a vinegar herbal extraction, and the second uses a vinegar reduction. To make an oxymel using a vinegar herbal extraction, use 1 part dried herb to 4 parts vinegar and honey. Put the mixture in a jar, seal it, store it in the dark, and shake it several times a week. After 2 to 3 weeks, strain and bottle it for use as needed.

If you're working with roots or in a rush, use a vinegar reduction: Add herbs and vinegar to a saucepan and heat on low. Let it reduce by half over 45 minutes on a low simmer. Once the liquid has cooled, add equal parts honey. This is a particularly palatable preparation and is easy to include in your daily diet.

---

#### → *Oxymel for Respiratory Health* ←

**MAKES ABOUT 1½ CUPS**

Combine 1 ounce each of dried rosemary, dried sage, and dried mullein flowers in an amber glass quart jar. Add 6 ounces each of apple cider vinegar and raw local honey. Stir well, place unbleached parchment paper as a barrier between the lid and the mouth of the jar (or use a plastic lid), then cover and let sit on a dark shelf, shaking daily. After 2 weeks, strain. Use 1 teaspoon every hour until respiration improves. Because oxymels are often needed in an emergency, like a sudden cold or bronchitis, it is best to prepare this well in advance.

---

## PLASTERS, POULTICES, AND RUBS

Herbal plasters, poultices, and rubs are meant to clear up congestion internally. They are usually applied to the chest to open up the respiratory passages but can also be applied to the lymph nodes to stimulate cleansing. Rubs tend to be diaphoretic and rubefacient in action. A rub is a must during a cold or pneumonia to mobilize waste, move lymph, and stimulate circulation. A traditional rub can speed the healing process and can be done daily until you feel better.

## SALVES

A salve is an external moisturizer made from herbal-infused oil and beeswax. Salves are helpful for musculoskeletal conditions or skin disorders. They tend to be solid at room temperature but soften with contact on the body. The infused oil is made from soaking herbal material in a shelf-stable carrier oil, like cold-pressed olive oil, coconut oil, or argan oil (*Argania spinosa*), or by heating the oil with plant material using a double boiler. Later, the menstruum is cooled and strained, and the oil with beeswax is added to the pan and heated just long enough for all the materials to blend and melt. The liquid is then poured into a container and left to cool. Salves tend to go rancid when left out in the sun or heat so be sure to store them in a cool place. Salves can also be made with bear fat or swine leaf lard. In Mexico, leaf lard is used topically as an anti-inflammatory and often with added basil, peyote, or cannabis to treat pain.

## SUPPOSITORIES

Suppositories are herbal preparations that are inserted rectally or vaginally. Suppositories are made by combining herbs with either an oily base like cocoa butter or a water-soluble substance like glycerin or gelatin and pouring it into premade molds. Another option is to combine finely powdered root, essentials oils, and coconut oil, roll pieces of it into appropriate sizes, and immediately place them in the freezer. Suppositories for the vagina can be used overnight with a sanitary pad. Rectal suppositories need to be inserted with immediate access to a toilet.

## SYRUPS

Syrups are essentially concentrated decoctions with honey or another liquid sweetener such as molasses. Syrups are tasty forms of medicine that are palatable to children and excellent remedies for sore throats or colds.

## TEA

Sometimes referred to as an infusion or tisane, a tea is an appropriate mode of preparation for leaves, flowers, and other delicate parts of plants. In an herbal tea, water is the solvent extracting the medicinal parts of herbs. Medicinal teas are typically stronger than regular teas. I recommend 1 part dried herb to 4 parts water or 1 part fresh plant material to 2 parts water. Medicinal teas may have a strong, bitter taste. Fill a jar with the herbal matter, pour hot water over it, and let the herbs soak for at least 30 minutes. Strain and enjoy. The tea will keep for 12 hours at room temperature or for 3 days in the fridge.

## TINCTURE

A tincture is a simple, long-lasting herbal preparation that uses a high-proof alcohol like ethanol to extract the medicinal compounds from the herbs and create a potent, liquid medicine. Ethanol is an excellent solvent for alkaloids and volatile oils, which are harder to extract with water. Among the alcohols I use to make tinctures are tequila, rum, and vodka, The essential requirement is to use a minimum of 80 proof alcohol to obtain the best results. Tinctures are especially handy for acute flare-ups and conditions. You can simply add a dropperful of a tincture to an ounce or two of water. An alcohol-based tincture would not be appropriate for those who cannot consume alcohol; instead try a glycerite or a vinegar extraction. Making a tincture requires soaking the herb in a strong spirit for at least 4 weeks in a dry, cool place, and later straining and bottling the material. An alcohol tincture tends to have a shelf life of 4 to 6 years.

## VAGINAL DOUCHE

A vaginal douche involves applying water or a water-and-vinegar-dilution-infused liquid into the vaginal canal and region for a rinse or cleanse. However, vaginas are self-cleansing, and current thinking suggests that douches should be avoided. A vaginal steam may be a healthier alternative (see below).

## VAGINAL STEAM

A vaginal or a yoni steam (yoni is the Hindu word for vulva) is a treatment using vapors from an herbal infusion to support vaginal health. Water and herbs are heated in a container over which you can sit or squat. This allows the steam to enter and surround the vagina. This process uses herbs known for their ability to strengthen and tonify the uterus and vaginal tissue. The vaginal garden is a self-cleansing mechanism and does not need cleaning per se, though it can get out of balance with bacterial or fungal infections. Steams are used to improve fertility and sexual sensitivity as well as to treat premenstrual syndrome (PMS), menstrual pain, and endometriosis.

# CONCLUSION

How we prepare herbs for prevention, treatment, and ritual uses influences their effects and how likely we are to use them consistently. We frequently know what we need or want to use as an herbal preparation and how often we want to use it, but our lifestyle or other social or health factors may get in the way of our actually applying our knowledge and using these medicines.

Learning which preparation methods work best for you and your family and knowing how herbs perform best can guide you in your healing discoveries. Over time, as your needs change or become more complex, how you prepare and use herbs may also change. Thus is the dynamic interaction between you and the gifts healing herbs bring.

## → 3 ←

# HERBS FOR DAY-TO-DAY HEALING AND SEASONAL RHYTHMS

One August Sunday in Mexico when the air was thick with moisture, and steam was rising from the heat of the ground, Señora Gorgonia rang the bell on my gate and invited me on a walk along with her mother, Doña Flavia. She said that they were going to swim out to *la punta*, the point of land that juts out into the sea, to pick herbs, and they would point out remedies along the way, if I wanted to join them. Before we left her house, Flavia pointed to a common plant called sin vergüenza (*Tradescantia zebrina*) meaning "shameless." She explained further that when mashed together with vinegar it relieves the swelling and pain of varicose veins, a serious problem for many women in the village. As we walked, Flavia picked and pulled at branches of *llantén* (plantain), whose leaves are commonly applied to a scorpion sting, only after you catch the scorpion and lay it on top of the sting, dead, of course. She drew my attention to delicate white flowers called arnica that when macerated in alcohol and applied to a bruise or sprain alleviated pain and swelling. As we continued, she pointed down at the path at one remedy that she didn't touch, but said, "Take two handfuls and rub it in your scalp daily. It will make your hair thick and cure those without any." She was pointing at cow dung—we all laughed.

We arrived at our swimming spot, and Flavia climbed a small hill to shake a papaya out of a tree. Because the ripened fruit is easy to digest, it is eaten when one is ill and nothing else can be eaten. But Flavia also said that the unripe fruit holds the strongest medicine. The milky substance between the skin and the fruit is an enzyme called papain. The villagers applied a slice of the skin to meat to soften it, to an infection to draw out the pus, or to a bee sting to soothe the pain. The papaya seeds can be dried and used as a medicinal tea to rid the bowels of parasites and worms. As we sat on the rocks soaking our feet in the cool water, clouds began to form overhead, and the *guacos* (laughing falcons) flew by laughing their unusual song. Flavia suggested that we start back, warning that I better get ready to pay off all my debts, because it looked as though it might begin to rain while the sun was still shining.

My walks with Flavia and Gorgonia continued over the years as they introduced me to a variety of herbs for everyday prevention and those reserved for specific illnesses. They shared with me both the art and science of indigenous ways of knowing: of how plants and animals reveal their medicines and the trial and error of preparation. They also introduced me to other herbalists and healers who had their own specialities and awakened in me a passion for listening deeply to the specific plants I needed as I traversed diverse geographies.

# WELCOME TO MY APOTHECARY

I always carry with me a basic herbal first aid kit, whether I am trekking in the forest or jungle or hopping on a plane to another country. Then, upon arrival in a new locale, I scout green and wild areas to learn more about where to plant my feet for health.

In this section I provide you with some instructions on how to create your own herbal first aid kit filled with herbs and medicines that you want to have available for emergencies and day-to-day healing needs. I also introduce you to many, many herbs along with recipes for their uses. You will learn about the specific ways that herbs keep us healthy, speed our healing when we are ill, or restore our balance after we recover.

## CREATE YOUR HERBAL
## MEDICINE CABINET AND FIRST AID KIT

One of the first things to do when you are starting your work with herbs is to make an herbal first aid kit filled with herbs and remedies that you want to have on hand all the time. It's a great way to access a wide range of remedies that will address the many health problems that can arise.

Making your own herbal first aid kit is a wonderful way to come into contact more deeply with healing plants, and it is a fun activity to share with children and friends. Gather together your friends and family to make salves or creams or have each person bring their favorite items (with instructions for use) to share with the group. Collect all your first aid essentials and pack them up in some favorite baskets or airtight boxes for the car, your home, and the office.

It's important to check the overall ingredients at least once a year to be sure they stay fresh. Some items, such as tea bags or loose herbs, should be checked every 6 months, while other ingredients like extracts and tinctures will last for up to 7 years. Capsules are an easy way to keep a variety of herbs in your kit. Store all herbs away from sunlight and in a cool place. I keep one of my boxes in the trunk of the car.

The following lists of tools, supplies, and herbal medicines and products will give you some ideas of what to include in your first aid kit to get you started. You can copy these pages and place them in your basket or plastic box as a checklist of sorts.

## TOOLS AND SUPPLIES

- Alcohol
- A range of adhesive bandages, gauze, and cotton balls
- 1 to 2 pounds of beach sand in an old pillow case
- 2 to 3 droppers or pipettes
- Hot water bottle (as a rule a hot water bottle is better than a heating pad, as it does not transmit the 60 Hz of electricity)
- Tweezers
- A small bottle of distilled water for drinking or wound cleansing

## HERBAL PRODUCTS

### TINCTURES

- Antispasmodic formula (available at Herb Pharm—see "Resources")
- California poppy tincture
- Kava tincture
- White willow tincture (or capsule)

### TEA BAGS/LOOSE HERBS

- Calendula tea bag
- Ground cayenne pepper in capsule or small bag

- Chamomile tea bag
- Licorice stick
- Meadowsweet tea bag
- Raspberry or blackberry leaf tea bag
- Slippery elm bark powder and/or lozenges
- Yarrow tea bag

**ESSENTIAL AND INFUSED OILS**

- Clove (*Syzygium aromaticum*) essential oil (or whole clove)
- Lavender essential oil
- Peppermint essential oil
- Rosemary essential oil
- Tea tree essential oil
- Cannabidiol (CBD) oil for topical or internal use
- Mullein garlic-infused oil

**SALVES**

- Arnica and comfrey salve
- Calendula salve
- Plantain salve

**OTHER ITEMS**

- Small bottle of aloe vera (*Aloe vera*) gel
- Bentonite clay and/or activated charcoal
- Chlorophyll tablets (or Gastrazyme) from Biotics Research, Inc.
- Ginger candies or extract
- A small bottle of witch hazel (*Hamamelis*) hydrosol

→ *Making Your Own Herbal Field Guide* ←

Herbalist Juliet Totten suggests creating your own field guide as a part of your first aid kit by selecting and focusing on useful plants in your own region. The field guide becomes personal to your lifestyle and the adventures you take. Researching the appearance and medicinal activity of each of the plants in greater depth will help you choose which ones you wish to include and help your ability to recognize them on your outdoor journeys.

Some suggestions of plants that will be especially important to know while in the field include dock (*Rumex crispus*), which is useful should you run into a patch of stinging nettle, jewelweed (*Impatiens capensis*), which will take the itch out of poison ivy (*Toxicodendron radicans*), plantain, which can be chewed and applied to bug bites, and yarrow leaves, which can quickly stop bleeding and a bloody nose.

## COMMON FIRST AID NEEDS AT HOME AND ON THE ROAD

Throughout this book, I have divided herbs into medicines and foods, and in the chapters that follow I address culinary spices and spirit herbs. These divisions are mostly arbitrary because herbs fulfill so many functions. What they do and how they work may just depend on the dose, the method of preparation, or even the reason for using them. Above all, the key is to find the many ways you can integrate herbs into your life and your home for pleasure, sustenance, and healing.

### ACUTE ANXIETY

The essential oil of lavender aromatherapy can be used in cases of acute anxiety; dabbing it on the temples and wrists is especially effective. A dropperful of kava or California poppy tincture will provide ease within 15 minutes in acute situations. Lastly, the underrated, but powerful, cup of chamomile tea is often the best way to combat anxiety.

### ALLERGIES

A tea of stinging nettle can be used to combat seasonal allergies. Echinacea is also useful as it works to modulate the hyperactive immune reaction, which causes inflammatory symptoms to flare in allergic reaction.

### ANTISPASMODIC

There are many emergency conditions that can lead to the need for an antispasmodic herb or compound. An antispasmodic, also called a spasmolytic, is useful for a range of problems including respiratory spasms (due to cough, bronchitis, or asthma), acute muscles spasms, menstrual cramps, bowel cramping (due to dysentery or food poisoning), migraines, bladder or ureter spasms (due to urinary tract infections), and hiccups. They can even be helpful if you are coming down with the flu.

Antispasmodic herbs to have on hand include hyssop, ephedra (ma huang) (*Ephedra sinica*), thyme, lobelia, passionflower, chamomile, and elecampane. Over the years I have relied on the formula proposed by herbalist Jethro Kloss that includes the following herbs: black cohosh root, myrrh resin, skullcap flowering tops, skunk cabbage root, lobelia in flower and seed form, and ground cayenne pepper. Herbalists Sara Katz and Ed Smith, at HerbPharm, make a wonderful version of this formula.

Immediately after administering the herbal medicine, perform the "Perineal Antispasmodic Relaxation Technique" (see below) to reduce spasms.

### ⇛ *Perineal Antispasmodic Relaxation Technique* ←

I have practiced this treatment, called the perineal rock, on thousands of clients and when combined with the herbal antispasmodic it provides profound relaxation and alleviation of symptoms. Perform this treatment just after giving the first dose of antispasmodic, while waiting for it to take effect. Use this in emergency situations when your patient is anxious or cannot sleep or to induce deep relaxation and release both physical and emotional tension.

This first phase involves contact with the sacrum and coccyx. The second phase requires direct contact with the perineum and underneath the coccyx. While you may do phase 2 on a family member, with permission, you will certainly want to assess whether you do it on anyone else in an emergency and only then with permission, since contact underneath the coccyx and perineum is a sensitive region. If you're doing this on a client, you should be trained and licensed to touch, and the client should feel comfortable with the intimate contact and give you permission to do it. Couples can learn to do this for each other in times of stress.

To begin, position the patient on her right side supported by a small pillow beneath her head and one between her knees. Sit or stand at her back and simultaneously place your right hand between the shoulder blades and your left hand on the sacrum. The sacrum is the triangular bone at the base of the spine, between the two hipbones. The word sacrum means sacred and is also considered a holy bone. In Hinduism, the Kundalini is the life force represented in the form of a coiled female snake who sleeps in the sacrum awaiting awakening through consciousness practices like meditation and yoga.

Begin rocking the sacrum while keeping the shoulder contact steady. The rocking is gentle, slow, and barely perceptible. Invite the patient to close her eyes and focus on a relaxed rhythm of breathing. If this method does not deliver complete results, try phase 3, which is called the Rectal Massage Technique (see page 225).

### ASTHMA ATTACK
See treatment under "Asthma" (page 199), with application of cold pack or ice pack. See also the antispasmodic herbs referred to in "Antispasmodic" (page 35) and the Perineal Antispasmodic Relaxation Technique (page 35).

### BLEEDING
Ground cayenne pepper or fresh yarrow leaf can be pressed directly into a wound, or nose, to arrest bleeding.

### BURNS
Aloe vera gel can be very useful for minor burns, as can an infusion of calendula or an oil infused with St. John's wort (which becomes the most beautiful red color), all of which work to soothe and heal the wound.

### CIRCULATION/CHILBLAINS
Ground cayenne pepper can be sprinkled into socks and gloves to encourage blood flow to hands and feet. Be careful not to rub your eyes!

### COLD/FLU
A warming drink combining the juice of a lemon or lime, some blackstrap molasses, and a pinch of ground cayenne pepper can be sipped slowly to ease a cold. Also see the suggestion for the Simple Garlic Onion Soup (page 76).

### DEHYDRATION
Licorice stick can be soaked in water or decocted and sipped as a cooling, hydrating remedy, which also helps to prevent heatstroke.

### DIARRHEA
An infusion of raspberry or blackberry leaf and/or meadowsweet can be especially useful for treating bouts of diarrhea. If the diarrhea is caused by intestinal worms, use an anthelmintic (see "Intestinal Helminths," page 38).

### EARACHE
Place your bottle of infused mullein and garlic oil in a pot of gently boiling water for a minute or two, then test a dot of the oil on the inside of the wrist to make sure it is not too hot. Administer 1 to 2 drops of warmed oil in each ear.

Earaches due to infection or sinus congestion also respond to onion-and-garlic soup. These sulfurous vegetables reduce infectious agents and break up mucus.

## FEVER

Yarrow tea can help to break a fever by encouraging perspiration, while white willow or a tea of meadowsweet can each be taken as a febrifuge, which helps reduce fever.

## GASTRITIS/GASTROESOPHAGEAL REFLUX DISEASE (GERD)

Drink two 8-ounce glasses of water upon awakening and drink 50 percent of your body weight in ounces throughout the day. Drink fresh cabbage juice taken with chlorophyll tablets (or try a pill that combines chlorophyll and vitamin U from cabbage). Slowly sip the juice or take 3 pills until symptoms abate.

## EXHAUSTION

See "Acute Anxiety" (page 34). The herbs suggested there can encourage a deep and healing sleep, the best remedy for when you are depleted and exhausted.

## HEADACHE

The essential oils of lavender and peppermint can be used to stop a headache as aromatherapy and/or applied directly to the temples. If peppermint is applied to the skin, it should first be diluted with a "carrier oil" such as apricot kernel (*Prunus armeniaca*) or jojoba (*Simmondsia chinensis*). The analgesic action of white willow, in capsule or tincture, or of meadowsweet in infusion, can also soothe a headache.

## HICCUPS (ACUTE AND CHRONIC)

See the antispasmodic herbs referred to in "Antispasmodic" (page 35) and the "Rectal Massage Technique" (page 225).

## INSECT BITES/STINGS

Plantain is known as the "Band-Aid plant" and also "white man's footstep" by natives of North America because the plant arrived and spread everywhere the Europeans seemed to go. Commonly found along roadsides, it makes an excellent emergency plant to be used topically; simply crush the fresh leaves of plantain and apply them directly to the bite to reduce inflammation and itching. It is also an edible leaf and can be eaten if you are out in the woods without food. A salve of plantain is useful when treating insect bites, as is lavender essential oil, which can be applied topically to reduce itching.

Slippery elm acts as a wonderful drawing salve when mixed with water to form a paste and applied to a bite or sting. If you have access to fresh green papaya, score the green skin; the white substance that emerges is papain and can be used directly on the sting or a wound. You can also keep some papain capsules on hand. You simply break them and apply the papain directly to a bee or wasp sting.

Use vitamin C powder, rosehips, or roselle (*Hibiscus sabdariffa*) internally to detoxify the venom from a bite or sting. High intravenous (IV) doses (50,000 to 100,000 milligrams) of vitamin C can be used in case of a venomous snakebite or scorpion sting while getting to urgent care, or 5,000 millgrams of oral vitamin C can be taken every hour.

### INTESTINAL HELMINTHS (PARASITES)

Combine back walnut with goldenseal and Oregon grape, or barberry and wormwood to make an effective antihelminthic. Garlic can also be useful if other remedies are unavailable.

### NAUSEA

Candied ginger and ginger extract are helpful in treating nausea and digestive upset and are very tasty. A tisane of meadowsweet can also be used.

### POISONING

It's always wise to have on hand both bentonite clay for food poisoning and activated charcoal for poisoning of any kind for children, adults, and animals.

Bentonite clay can be stored as a powder or a liquid and taken internally (½ cup). In the case of poisoning or an aspirin overdose, emergency help should be sought immediately, but in the meantime one can take activated charcoal but only after speaking to the poison control center.

---

### » Oral Dose of Activated Charcoal to Treat Poisoning «

Treatment with one dose:

- Adults and teenagers: Dose is usually 25 to 100 grams mixed with water.
- Children 1 through 12 years of age: Dose is usually 25 to 50 grams mixed with water, or the dose may be based on body weight. It may be 0.5 to 1 gram per kilogram (0.23 to 0.45 grams per pound) of body weight mixed with water.
- Children up to 1 year of age: Dose is usually 10 to 25 grams mixed with water, or the dose may be based on body weight. It may be 0.5 to 1 gram per kilogram (0.23 to 0.45 grams per pound) of body weight mixed with water.

---

### SHOCK

While waiting for help to arrive, rosemary essential oil as aromatherapy can help to stabilize someone who is in shock or has been acutely traumatized.

### SLEEP AIDE

A passionflower tincture is especially beneficial for those who are struggling to get to sleep and stay asleep. The herbs used for acute anxiety also encourage deep, restful sleep and relaxation.

### SPRAINS, STRAINS, AND BRUISES

The first step in treating a strain, sprain, or bruise is R-I-C-E, meaning: Rest, Ice, Compress, and Elevate. Use RICE for at least the first 48 to 72 hours after an injury. At the same time, for the first 48 to 72 hours avoid H-A-R-M, which stands for Heat, Alcohol, Exercise, and Massage. All of these can increase swelling and bleeding, which slow healing.

Apply arnica and comfrey salve to sprains and bruises. Fresh crushed plantain or the bruised leaves of comfrey may also be applied externally.

Quercetin-rich foods, like apples, berries, cherries, and parsley, should be eaten (with oil for absorption). Try a smoothie with a dollop of coconut cream or oil. These plants and fruits are natural anti-inflammatories and help restore blood vessel integrity, especially in bruising.

After 48 to 72 hours of RICE, apply the following herbal hot sand recipe to a sprain that will top off the whole treatment.

---

→ *Treatment of Sprain with Arnica and Sand* ←

Lightly rub arnica salve all around the ankle, wrist, or sprained joint. Take 1 to 2 pounds of sand from the beach and put it inside a small pillowcase. Place it in a baking dish and heat at 350°F for 20 minutes. When it has cooled enough to apply, place the bag so that the sand covers the whole ankle. The minerals from the sand will penetrate and help heal the ankle more quickly. Do this treatment 3 times a day for 3 days.

---

### STOMACHACHE. *See also* "Nausea" (page 38).

An infusion of chamomile tea always helps, and this is especially true in cases of stomach upset. Acting as a gentle bitter, chamomile aids digestion, and its relaxing nervine qualities ease spasms throughout the gastrointestinal tract.

### SUNBURN

A few drops of rose oil added to almond oil soothes a sunburn.

### TOOTHACHE

Clove oil can be rubbed directly on the painful tooth, or alternatively one can lightly bite down on a whole clove.

### VAGINAL INFECTION

Prick a clove of garlic with a needle a few times to release its constituents and then sew a string through the clove (which is to be used as a suppository) so it can be easily removed.

A sitz (hip) bath of strong calendula tea can also be used in cases of fungal (yeast) infection and in cases of general vaginal discomfort.

### WOUND HEALING

Mix slippery elm powder with water to form a poultice to remove debris and dead tissue from a wound. Then apply an infusion or salve of calendula as a vulnerary to speed healing. A witch hazel hydrosol can be used as an antiseptic to cleanse the wound, and if desired, other herbs such as calendula or a few drops of tea tree oil can be added to make it an even more powerful healing agent. Garlic is also a potent antimicrobial, but it can burn the skin if left on too long when applied directly, so use with caution.

## THE RHYTHMS OF WOMEN'S HEALTH

Balancing the rhythms of our bodies and minds is one of the most important foundations for our health. Herbs are uniquely suited to help us with this as they have their own internal clock, regulated by the light and dark, and grow in response to nature's rhythms, storing nourishment that furthers our own rhythms. For example, licorice root regulates the rhythms of the stress response in the brain, hawthorn enhances the muscle contractions of the heart, and my favorite drink, Jamaica, reduces pressure on arterial rhythms and lowers blood pressure as a result.

When we get out of rhythm, we feel "out of sync," "beside ourselves," or "off kilter." Nature, through the daily cycle of light and dark, through photosynthesis of plants with the light-giving molecules of chlorophyll, entrains us to our biological cycles. These cycles include the circadian rhythm of our 24-hour sleep-wake cycle, the 120-minute cycle of brain hemispheric dominance, and the monthly cycle of our egg release and menstrual flow. The 24-hour sleep-wake cycle regulates hormonal responses that govern mood, sleep, and reproductive health including fertility and menstruation.

Fertility, bowel movements, blood pressure, and even our risk of dementia are also governed by circadian rhythm and herbs help us to align with these rhythms.

Understanding the role of these rhythms on our well-being provides us with insight into how modern life, travel across time zones, working the "graveyard shift," and the ways chronic stress turn our clock around affect each of our life stages, whether we are trying to ease menstrual flow, get pregnant, or navigate the surges of menopause.

Let's begin by honoring our seasonal rhythms with special detoxification rituals that align our bodies and minds to the rhythms of nature each season.

## SPRING CLEANSE

There is no better annual herbal ritual than spring-cleaning. After a winter of hibernation, our organs, inside and out, benefit from cleansing and purification. Nature provides us with the plants that pop in the spring so we can nourish and cleanse our organs. After all, we change our car's oil filter and take it in for a lube and wash. Why not do the same for our internal organs?

→ *Morning Liver Flush* ←

**MAKES 1 SERVING**

This liver flush is designed to be done for 10 days and consists of this juice recipe and the following Ayurvedic Polarity Tea and Liver Cleanse Menu. Make both drinks each morning and alternate sips until finished, then follow with your first meal an hour later. This cleanse could also be conducted if you are diagnosed with stones and wish to avoid surgery.

Take 6 to 8 ounces of freshly squeezed citrus juice (orange, grapefruit, lime) and add 1 to 2 tablespoons of virgin cold-pressed olive oil and 1 thumb of fresh ginger. Combine in a blender. Make and drink this tea every morning, waiting 1 hour after drinking it before having breakfast.

## » *Ayurvedic Polarity Tea* «

This Ayurvedic recipe supports the liver, gallbladder, and adrenal glands, aids digestion, enhances energy, reduces allergic reactions, and is soothing to respiratory and intestinal mucous membranes. It acts as a mild laxative and stimulant. The recommended dose is 1 cup of tea per day along with the Morning Liver Flush.

**MAKES 5 OUNCES DRIED MIX, 10 SERVINGS**

1 ounce licorice root pieces

1 ounce fenugreek seed

1 ounce fennel seed

2 ounces flaxseed

Mix all the dry ingredients together and store the mixture in a glass jar in a dark cabinet until you need it. Take 1 heaping tablespoon of the mixture and simmer in 2 cups of boiling water until it is reduced to 1 cup or so, 15 to 20 minutes. Strain and drink hot in the morning.

## LIVER CLEANSE MENU

For 10 days, eat only raw and cooked vegetables, topped with the bitter herbs of spring such as fresh dandelions or arugula. Top the raw and cooked vegetables with a dressing of virgin cold-pressed olive oil, lemon, garlic, and lots of fresh herbs like dill, basil, and oregano. Eat plenty of beets and beet greens. Eat as much as you want and as often as you want but only fresh vegetables and fruits and the dressing. At the end of 10 days, slowly integrate your regular food back into your menu.

## » *Beets and Beet Greens* «

Beets and beet greens are rich in betaine, which stimulates the flow of bile and supports detoxification. When you buy beets try to find them with fresh greens still attached. Steam the beets with the jackets on for 45 to 60 minutes, depending on their size. Don't poke them while cooking as the juices will be lost. Serve them hot or cold with sea salt, or put them in a blender and make a beet soup. The greens make a wonderful stir-fry with onions and garlic, all of which detoxify the liver and boost the mood.

## ↠ *Coffee Enema* ↞

One of the most effective ways to benefit from coffee is via an enema. In contrast to the effects of drinking coffee, which stimulates the adrenal glands, coffee enemas provide a type of dialysis of the liver and support what is called phase two detoxification. As the major detoxifying organ, the liver has two phases of releasing toxins that must pass out of the body. The first phase breaks down these toxins using the P450 enzyme process. P450 may sound familiar because many herbs I discuss in the book interact with the P450 enzyme process and thereby may speed or slow elimination of medications or toxins.

Phase two takes over to further break down the toxins and is enhanced by the foods, herbs, and nutrients we ingest. This is where the coffee enema plays a role because it enhances the phase two process. Coffee enemas are also used in the treatment of cancer pain and, unlike the effects felt from drinking coffee, the enemas are actually very relaxing. The detoxification process is not about emptying the lower part of the colon, though that is a side benefit; the enema also helps to release bile. Coffee enemas can be done daily or if in pain or very toxic, twice a day, or you might begin with a few times a week.

You will need a colon tube for this enema. Colon tubes are identified by length of the tube and the size (diameter of the tube) (French size). I recommend a 20-inch-long, size 28 French. Prepare a comfortable place in your bathroom. This might include a thick rug covered with a towel and a pillow for resting your head. (Once you are able to control the retention of the fluid, you may "fill up" in the bathroom and then make a place on your bed, covered with a towel, where you may rest during the enema.) Once they have mastered the process, people tell me they listen to a podcast, chat on the phone with a friend, watch a video, get some reading done, or rest and meditate during the enema.

Prepare a quart of organic coffee, using 2 tablespoons of coffee grounds per quart of nonchlorinated water. The water should be purified and not taken from the tap unless it is first filtered. Decaffeinated coffee will not work for enemas. Decaf does not contain the cafestol (a compound found in Arabica coffee beans) required to effect the liver cleansing. The coffee should be made in a stainless steel or glass coffee maker. Aluminum is not recommended, and do not use paper filters as they will filter out the cafestrol. "Cowgirl coffee" is an easy way to make your enema preparation. You can add 1 teaspoon of unsulfured blackstrap molasses to each quart of coffee, while the coffee is hot, if you have trouble retaining the enemas. Make sure you judge the ratios correctly to maintain the correct strength. For efficiency, make a quart of this coffee mixture in advance and keep it in the fridge. Then keep an electric pot in the bathroom to heat up water as needed. The coffee is best used at body temperature.

When preparing to take the enema, lie on your left side, and lubricate the colon tube and the anus using a lubricant like K-Y jelly. Insert the colon tube slowly 12 to 18 inches (never more than 18) into the rectum. Release the stopper and let about a pint of coffee slowly flow in, then clamp down again. Take in a little liquid and release immediately in the toilet to flush out collected waste in the rectum. This allows for easier retention. At first, it may be difficult to retain the enema. If this is the case begin with half a cup and increase the amount as you get used to the process. Retain the coffee for 10 minutes before expelling. Do not hold the enemas for longer than 15 minutes. Repeat the enema, holding for another 10 minutes. Do 2 doses, each consisting of 1 pint held for 10 minutes, in the morning. Do not do enemas after 3:00 PM. as they can be stimulating later into the evening.

If after the first few sessions you feel jittery or have trouble falling asleep, you are making the coffee too strong. For best results do the coffee enema daily. A coffee enema can be done in 25 minutes from start to finish once you get the routine in place. Make it part of your overall self-care routine.

---

## CLEANING OUR HOMES

While we are cleaning our insides, we can take some time to use herbs to cleanse our environment as well. Exposure to toxins can be dangerous for all of us, but especially during pregnancy and the first few years of life as the nervous system is developing. We cannot eliminate all exposure, but we can reduce our risk. Start with your cleaning products and soaps and eliminate all pesticides or fertilizers. If you cannot buy all organic foods, detoxify fruits and vegetables prior to consumption. The most toxic fruits and vegetables, however, should always be organic. They include celery, spinach, potatoes, apples, grapes, and peaches. To eliminate pesticides and fertilizers from produce, fill a sink with water, add 3 cups of water, 1 cup of vinegar, and 5 drops of lemon essential oil. Let the vegetables and fruits soak for 5 minutes, then wash, rinse, and dry thoroughly. Look underneath your sink and in your garage for toxic cleaning supplies, as well as drain and oven cleaners. If you have bought cleaning supplies in the store, they will likely be toxic. Throw them out and try the following healthy cleaning solution instead.

> ↠ *Healthy Cleaning Solution* ↞

Essential oils added to apple cider vinegar can take the place of harsh chemicals for cleaning. Add 10 drops of essential oils of tea tree, peppermint, lemon, or cinnamon to a quart of vinegar. This mixture can be used to clean dishes, counters, floors, toilets, and tubs. If you need to scrub, just make a paste of 3 parts baking soda to 1 part salt and add 10 drops of oil to it.

> ↠ *Cleanse the Home of Smells, Moths, and Bugs—Inside and Out!* ↞

Burning lemongrass and dried rosemary bundles can cleanse the home of any unwanted smells, and the potent volatile oils in lemongrass and rosemary prove offensive bugs. I also gather Mexican cinnamon and simmer a few pieces in water to create a lovely smell in my home, especially before greeting guests.

## SUMMER CLEANSE

Summer is the time to eliminate heavy metals that are stored in our fat. The heat of the season helps us build up a good sweat that eliminates the metals from our body that we have collected from breathing the air, eating, or walking on pesticides. This is a good time to sweat out your waste with a hard aerobic walk in the morning or early evening. Toxins like cadmium, lead, and mercury accumulate in tissues when protein is deficient in the diet. Sulfur is necessary for the process of detoxification. The sulfur compounds in proteins (sulfur-rich plants include garlic and onions), along with the cruciferous vegetables like cabbage, broccoli, and Brussels sprouts, protect the cells from heavy metal toxicity. Coriander, also known as cilantro or Chinese parsley, is another powerful antioxidant that removes heavy metals from the body.

Seaweed is one of the most important detoxifying foods because alginates from the brown seaweeds bind toxic metals and radioactive isotopes in the digestive tract. Seaweeds (particularly kelp with its natural sodium alginate compound built in) are a significant detoxifying food source. Adding seaweed to soups or bean dishes or eating it as a snack is healthy for the thyroid. Another option for this summer detox is to obtain sodium alginate that combines brown seaweeds and modified citrus pectin and take 3 capsules a day for 5 days in between meals.

Each day for 10 days, include a variety of seaweeds in your meals and emphasize the cruciferous and sulfuric plants. Sweat out your waste with a hard aerobic walk in the morning or early evening. Do coffee enemas (see page 43) daily to help move the waste through the liver and colon, and at night, just before bed, take milk thistle to support your liver overnight as it cleanses. After this easy detox you will be ready to frolic during the summer months.

## » *Starter Seaweed Salad Detox* «

I have designed this delicious seaweed salad to include the major detox plants from land and sea using arame sea vegetables, which are among the mildest of seaweeds. This salad is a good first step in exploring seaweeds in recipes.

**SERVES 6 TO 8**

1 cup dry arame seaweed

3 scallions, diced

1 cup carrots, diced

½ cup pea pods, diced

½ red bell pepper, diced

½ English cucumber, diced

Handful of broccoli florets, cut into
   bite-size pieces

¼ cup chopped walnuts or pine nuts

Clover sprouts

¼ cup chopped cilantro

**DRESSING**

¼ cup toasted sesame oil

¼ cup rice wine vinegar

1 tablespoon wheat-free tamari

1 clove garlic, finely chopped

1 thumb fresh ginger, finely chopped

Dash of hot red pepper flakes (optional)

Soak the seaweed in warm water for 15 minutes until soft (save the water for soup or to put in your animal companion's bowl). Combine the scallions, carrots, pea pods, red pepper, cucumber, broccoli, nuts, and sprouts in a bowl. In a separate bowl, add all of the dressing ingredients together and whisk until well combined. Combine the vegetable mixture with the softened seaweed and pour the dressing over it. Mix well and allow to marinate for a few hours. Top with cilantro before serving and enjoy!

## AUTUMN CLEANSE

Autumn is the transitional season between the summer light and the settling in of the deep winter dark. We are moving into the bowels of the year, and it's a good time to cleanse our own, even as we keep our mood bright. This colon cleanse celebrates our capacity to absorb, digest, and release, both literally and metaphorically.

### PSYLLIUM FLUSH

Three times a day, between each meal, mix a tablespoon of psyllium husk powder in 8 ounces of water. Stir and let sit for a minute, then drink it down and follow it with another 4 to 8 ounces of water. Do this cleanse for 5 days.

This is a 2-part cleanse. After the 5 days of psyllium flushing, ask family members or a gaggle of girlfriends to join you and celebrate your final day—with tea and prunes (recipe follows).

→ *Lapsang Souchong Tea and Prunes* ←

What could be better to lift one's spirits than a little caffeine as the sun starts to set combined with a relaxed, efficient release of old waste? My friend and super chef Peggy Knickerbocker developed this recipe, and I have adapted it here. It combines prunes, Armagnac (a brandy similar to cognac), and Lapsang souchong tea. Lapsang souchong is a smoky black tea with moderate caffeine content, and prunes are well known for their laxative effect. The touch of Armagnac adds an elegant and restful element.

SERVES 4 TO 6

1 pound pitted prunes

Zest of ½ large orange

1 thumb fresh ginger, unpeeled

2 cups Lapsang souchong, Earl Grey, or
 other hot brewed tea

10 drops stevia or 1 tablespoon raw local
 honey

Juice of 1 large orange

2 cinnamon sticks

½ cup Armagnac or cognac (optional)

1 cup crème fraîche or Greek yogurt

Put the prunes, orange zest, and ginger in a nonreactive saucepan and pour the tea over them. Soak for at least 1 hour or overnight. Pour off ⅔ cup of the tea from the prunes. Add the stevia, orange juice, cinnamon sticks, and Armagnac, if using. Turn on the heat and simmer over low heat for 10 to 15 minutes. Remove the ginger. Spoon the prunes into small bowls and serve with a dab of crème fraîche on top.

## WINTER CLEANSE

Winter brings the rhythm of rest; as nature darkens the light our physical and emotional roots sink into the earth, to prepare for the renewal spring will soon bring. During our hibernation our task is to cleanse simply and only as needed, when our immune system needs some fire to burn off the blahs brought by colds and infections. There is no better way to stimulate the immune system than the Hot Cure.

### ↠ Caliente Curación *(the Hot Cure) a.k.a. Fire Cider* ↞

At the start of every winter season I make a fresh batch of fire cider to have on hand in case of a cold or sinus congestion. Cleansing in advance can often stave off infections. Formulated and popularized by herbalist Rosemary Gladstar, this cocktail can be added to vinaigrettes and used on salads. In some people nightshades (*Solanaceae*) cause joint stiffness. If you are sensitive to the effects of nightshades, eliminate the cayenne pepper and jalapeños and add a bit more ginger.

See also Children's Caliente Popsicles for a Sore Throat on page 198 for an adaptation of this recipe that children can suck on when they are fighting a cold, flu, bronchitis, or pneumonia.

**MAKES ABOUT 4 CUPS**

½ cup freshly grated ginger
½ cup grated fresh horseradish root
    or ground horseradish
1 medium onion, chopped
10 cloves garlic, chopped
2 jalapeño peppers, chopped
1 tablespoon ground beetroot
Zest and juice of 1 lemon

Several sprigs fresh rosemary
1 tablespoon ground turmeric
¼ teaspoon ground cayenne pepper
1 tablespoon peppercorns
12 ounces apple cider vinegar or
    pineapple vinegar
¼ cup raw local honey

Put everything except the vinegar and honey in an amber glass quart jar. Add the vinegar and fill to an inch below the top. Shake well. Store in a dark, cool place for a month and shake daily. After 1 month, use cheesecloth to strain out the pulp, and pour the vinegar into a clean jar. Squeeze as much of the liquid as you can from the pulp while straining. Add the honey. Take it 1 tablespoon at a time, up to 3 tablespoons a day if ill or congested with allergic rhinitis, or mix ¼ cup with ¼ cup of virgin cold-pressed olive oil for a salad dressing.

## CONCLUSION

Some herbs are meant to be used daily to nourish our energy, boost our strength, or to treat a chronic imbalance. We might take a shot of specially tinctured herbs for a week to prevent an illness or prepare an herbal elixir for a seasonal cleanse. Whatever reason we might require an herb, when we reach out to nature, she provides numerous and diverse opportunities to benefit from and revel in her healing gifts.

# » 4 «

# HERBAL MEDICINES FOR EVERYDAY USE AND SPECIAL PURPOSES

I n this chapter I provide a review of herbs and background on their uses, applications, and appropriate doses for many of the herbs. I include the common name and their Latin classification so you can investigate the plants further because in practice, different herbs may be called the same name but in fact be a different plant. Some of the herbs I discuss in other chapters also appear here, but this chapter is your go-to resource when you want to know what herb is good for what purpose. Remember, while I may mention some special contraindications, every herb should always be explored for appropriate use during pregnancy, while nursing, and while taking other medications.

## » *Understanding Liquid Doses* «

When you see the recommended dosage and preparation instructions for herbs, you may be wondering, what does it all mean? Typically, it will say something like: fresh *Lavandula angustifolia* 1:2 (95%).

Here, *1:2* refers to the weight to volume ratio of the medicine. This means for every one part herb, also called the marc (weight in grams), there will be two parts of menstruum (volume in milliliters). The menstruum is the liquid (alcohol, vinegar, glycerine, etc.) that is being used to extract the herb's constituents. In this example, one part lavender at 10 grams would require 2 parts alcohol (20 milliliters). The percentage, in this case *95%*, refers to the percentage of alcohol that is being used for the extraction.

Each herb has a ratio and percentage that is optimal for extracting its constituents based on its solubility. Additionally, fresh herbs have different ratios than their dried counterparts due to higher water content and variations in solubility.

## USE YOUR SENSORY KNOWLEDGE

Herbs tell us a lot about how they will help us by their color and their tastes, so smelling, chewing, and salivating over bark and berries, leaves and roots invites your sensory knowledge. This is called organoleptic research and is often used in reference to herbal medicine. *Organoleptic* means "involving the use of one's sense organs." In herbalism this refers to employing the senses—taste, touch, sight, and smell—to more deeply understand a plant's medicine. Of these senses, taste can often provide the most insight into the action of an herbal medicine as well as the constituents within a plant. For example, a puckering feeling in the mouth when tasting an herb, akin to the one that comes from drinking a glass of red wine, indicates a plant's astringent contracting qualities. Herbs that are highly flavorful and aromatic in quality, such as lavender, mint, or basil, signal that they are high in volatile oils.

Organoleptic analysis can also give us insight into the quality of the herbs we are using. For example, when we bite into a high-quality echinacea root or chew on some kava root, our mouth should have a numb, tingling feeling. If this doesn't occur you may be tasting an herb that is old or of inferior quality, and thus not as medicinally active or beneficial.

In the following list, you will see that in most instances I describe the plant and provide its characteristic active compounds along with occasional cultural references to the herb's ancient uses. I concentrate on herbs that are important to our health as women. You will note that some herbs have been used historically as abortifacients, to induce abortion. I provide this information for general knowledge as well as to promote awareness of what *not* to use during pregnancy. It is well established that a medical abortion in a clinic is much safer than an herbal abortion, and I would never recommend using herbs for abortion.

# HERB LIST

This is not an exhaustive list of herbs, but I have chosen what I believe to be the most important, wide-ranging, and accessible ones. I also introduce you to some unusual ones that may be new to your home pharmacy. Please feel free to further investigate any herbs that interest you. I provide suggestions on dosing herbs based on a range of traditional herbal practices (indigenous sciences) and standardized biomedical science. This is meant only as a guide since dosing will depend on the individual, their health and weight, whether the herb is fresh or dry, and the proposed use.

### AGRIMONY, TALL HAIRY AGRIMONY
**(*Agrimonia eupatoria*; *Agrimonia gryposepala*)**
Agrimony is an herbaceous flowering perennial that is a part of the *Rosaceae* family. Common agrimony is native to Europe, and tall hairy agrimony is native to North America. All parts of the plant are used for medicinal purposes, including the burrs, which contain the seeds. Agrimony has been regarded as a powerful magic herb, used to ward off hexes, cure illness, and bring about a deep sleep when put under the pillow. It is an astringent herb, rich in tannins, which can make it useful as a tonic for the digestive system and for the kidneys and liver, as well as a muscle relaxant and a diuretic. The gallotannins and gallic acid contribute to the astringent properties of the plant that make it useful as a styptic, which is a common use by the Potawatomi people. The Cherokee use an infusion of the burrs as a febrifuge, antidiarrheal, and emmenagogue, and the Iroquois use the plant to stop diarrhea and vomiting in children. It is renowned as a vulnerary and a hypoglycemic treatment for type 2 diabetes. Pour 1 cup of boiled water over 2 teaspoons of fresh or dried mix of leaves and flowers, Let sit for 15 minutes and strain. Drink 1 to 2 cups daily. If using topically as a vulnerary, let cool and rinse your wound or apply a compress of the tea.

### ALFALFA (*Medicago sativa*)
Alfalfa is a leguminous, perennial flowering herb native to West Asia. It has a very deep taproot that often reaches six feet into the soil. Alfalfa is highly effective as a nitrogen fixer, which means it draws nitrogen from the atmosphere to serve as a natural land fertilizer. The saponins in the alfalfa help to prevent heart disease by inhibiting cholesterol from attaching to arterial walls, and the isoflavones are especially useful for women's hormone balance and are used to prevent osteoporosis and the vasomotor effects (hot flashes) associated with menopause. Rich in vitamin K,

alfalfa helps to prevent blood clots and plays a central role in bone formation, making it essential for menopausal women. Alfalfa is rich in minerals, such as calcium, vitamins C and B, and antioxidants and is often combined with chlorophyll extract to provide a restorative tonic to aid digestion and the recovery from malnutrition. It is also rich in iron and thus improves hemoglobin function and is a natural approach to addressing anemia. The sprouted seeds of the alfalfa plant are easy to grow and a fun way to teach young children about plant growth. Take 1 teaspoon of dried alfalfa leaf and pour over 1½ cups of boiling water. Let steep for 15 minutes, strain, and drink. Make a cup daily for 1 week, then rotate in other herbs before returning to alfalfa 3 weeks later.

### ↠ *Menopausal Tea* ↞

A delicious, enriching tea for perimenopausal and menopausal symptoms can be made from 1 ounce each of alfalfa, nettle leaf, red clover flowers (*Trifolium pratense*), and horsetail. Mix the dried ingredients together and store in an amber glass jar. Make a tea by taking 1 tablespoon of the dry herb mix and pouring over 1½ cups of boiling water. Let sit for 15 minutes, strain, and drink. This brew can alkalinize the body pH, so drink it for 1 week out of the month only.

### ALOE VERA (*Aloe vera*)

Aloe vera is a flowering succulent commonly used as a topical and internal remedy. So revered is this plant for the good luck and healing it brings that it is called the Wand of Heaven and is frequently found at entranceways to homes or shops throughout Mexico. Aloe's gel is an anti-inflammatory and helps to heal burns. Whether you keep a plant inside or outside it should be close to your kitchen in case of a cooking burn. Aloe contains aloin, which is a laxative, and while some people ingest aloe vera gel for this purpose, it is best used as a topical agent. Better laxative choices would include short-term use of senna or cascara sagrada.

### ANGELICA (*Angelica; Angelica archangelica*)

Angelica, also called wild celery, is an aromatic flowering plant that belongs to the parsley family. While all parts of the plant are used, the root and rhizome are where most of the active ingredients are found, particularly blood-thinning coumarin derivatives. Angelica is used as a digestive aid for heartburn, intestinal gas, and loss of appetite. It can be used as an emmenagogue to increase urine production and to improve libido. It is also an excellent respiratory herb to be used as an expectorant for colds, congestion, and fevers.

Angelica has a rich history in northern European folklore as a cure-all and a protector against spells and enchantments as well as contagion. The Sámi people in Scandinavia regard it as a shamanic herb, and in Germany it is a main ingredient in digestifs to drink during and after a rich meal. To make a decoction, simmer 1,500 milligrams of root in 1 cup of water for 15 minutes, strain, and drink twice a day as needed.

CAUTION: Avoid excess sun exposure while using angelica as it can cause inflammation.

### ARNICA (*Arnica*; *Arnica montana*)

A perennial alpine wildflower, *Arnica montana* is the best-known species of arnica used for medicinal purposes. Arnica is frequently applied externally in salves and ointments for all sorts of aches and pains. It is a popular ingredient used in sports-related injuries, carpel tunnel syndrome, and arthritis, as well as for poor circulation. It may be paired with calendula to treat bruising. Do not use arnica internally as helenalin, which is a compound found in both arnica flowers and rhizomes that acts as an anti-inflammatory and antiseptic, can be toxic. I suggest oral homeopathic arnica as a safe internal adjunct.

### ARTICHOKE (*Cynara scolymus*)

The globe artichoke is a well-known edible flower in the thistle family. Like its milk thistle cousin, the fresh leaves of the young plant are strongly diuretic and work well in a liver tonic. Artichokes are a medicinal food high in antioxidants and the prebiotic inulin so beneficial for the intestines. Cynarine, a bitter-tasting compound in the leaves, improves liver and gallbladder functions, stimulates the secretion of gastric juices, reduces heartburn symptoms, lowers high cholesterol, and improves symptoms of irritable bowel syndrome (IBS). Artichoke is the principal flavoring in the liquor Cynar, usually served as an aperitif or digestif.

---

### ⟶ *Artichokes for the Heart* ⬅

Artichokes are a fun food to share around the table, and the leaves, along with this dipping sauce, are medicine for the heart. They have a delicate flavor and make a good food for a ritual or party.

**ARTICHOKES:** I prefer to steam artichokes rather than boil them. Take sharp scissors and snip off the prickly end of the artichokes. Then place the trimmed flower in a large steamer pot. Let the flower steam until you can pull the leaves off easily and they are tender when you run your teeth over them to loosen the pulp (about 45 minutes of hard steam).

**DIPPING SAUCE:** There are many dipping sauces for artichokes available, but this simple one is quick, easy, and medicinal. Warm ½ cup of ghee in a saucepan. Add 10 garlic cloves, adding some tarragon or cayenne pepper if you like, and let simmer until the garlic is cooked (10 to 15 minutes). When the garlic is done, pour it into a dipping bowl, serve it with the artichokes, and start dipping!

When you get down to the choke (the inedible fuzzy center) pull it out, cut off the fuzzy hair, and then drop the heart in the warm ghee and garlic. **NOTE:** Don't be afraid of ghee! It's good for your arteries, as is the garlic, so all three main ingredients support cholesterol and heart health.

---

### ASHWAGANDHA (*Withania somnifera*)

Ashwagandha is an herb I always want to have on hand. It is one of the most important adaptogens and an Ayurvedic treatment for chronic stress and fatigue. *Ashwagandha* means "the smell and strength of a horse," which is suggestive of its power. It contains withanolides (a group of flavonoids), which have steroidal effects in the body. I use ashwagandha to provide support when I'm stressed, and I will use it if I have a period of strenuous labor ahead of me, so that I am prepared and have the endurance I need. Traditionally, both the root and berries are used, though the root holds most of the medicinal properties. In Ayurvedic medicine, ashwagandha is always used in combination with other herbs as part of adaptogenic and general tonic formulas. It is a mild sedative and an aphrodisiac with no reported side effects.

Ashwagandha improves memory, stabilizes mood, and helps withdrawal from addictive substances. It also increases the libido, reduces inflammation, and helps to normalize sleep. The powder from the ground-up root of ashwagandha can be applied topically to swelling, boils, or arthritic joints and mixed into food, like my Ashwaganda Power Balls (recipe follows).

## ↠ Ashwagandha Power Balls ↞

Power balls are a great way to take your medicine, whether you are tired of swallowing capsules, would rather eat your herbs, or need a way to get your children to take some of the bitter herbs that are so medicinal.

Power balls make healthy treats, and you will feel virtuous getting your energizing herbs as a dessert or a snack. You can freeze them in small bags and just grab 1 to 2 a day as needed. The ingredients you can use in these balls are versatile, so feel free to experiment. In this recipe for 8 balls, 1 heaping teaspoon of ashwagandha powder is an appropriate dose for 4 days, if you eat 2 balls a day.

**MAKES 8 BALLS**

½ cup ground fresh coconut (do not use presweetened coconut)

3 teaspoons almond butter

3 teaspoons raw local honey

3 teaspoons cocoa powder

1 teaspoon bee pollen

3 teaspoons chia seed

⅓ cup raw sunflower seeds

1 heaping teaspoon ashwagandha powder

Begin by toasting the coconut over low heat in a cast-iron skillet until lightly browned, stirring to avoid burning. Set aside to cool. Add the almond butter to a large mixing bowl along with all the other ingredients one by one, stirring and mixing. As you add ingredients the mixture will become thicker, and you will have to knead it to blend the ingredients. Drop the dough onto a sheet of wax paper and knead it like bread dough for about 5 minutes. Roll the dough into a log about ¾ of an inch thick and, beginning at one end of the wax paper, roll the log several times, wrapping it in the wax paper as you go. Then roll the log back again, peeling off the wax paper. Cut the log into 8 equal pieces and roll each piece into a firm ball. Then press and roll each ball in the toasted coconut. Set aside in a dish in the fridge and enjoy 1 to 2 balls a day. They will be edible for months but you will gobble them up before a month goes by!

## ASTRAGALUS (*Astragalus propinquus*)

*Astragalus* is the largest genus of flowering plants. The roots of *Astragalus membranaceus* are rich in saponins, flavonoids, and polysaccharides, which give the herb its antioxidative, anti-inflammatory, and immune-boosting qualities. The dried root of the astragalus plant is referred to as *huang qi* in Chinese medicine and is used to increase vitality and, when combined with ginseng, to reduce fatigue. It is also adaptogenic and helps to prevent colds and upper respiratory illnesses.

## → *Immune Support Soup* ←

This soup will give you an important immune system boost to prevent a cold or reduce stress that may make you vulnerable to illness. Visit an Asian grocery store or Chinese herbal clinic and purchase some fresh or dried astragalus root to add to a soup. Be sure to remove it before eating the soup.

**SERVES 4**

6 cups freshly made chicken (or vegetable) broth

¼ cup astragalus root

1 carrot, diced

1 sweet potato, diced

1 zucchini, diced

2 celery stalks, sliced

1 onion, diced

2 cloves garlic, crushed

1 thumb fresh ginger

Handful of reishi or shiitake mushrooms

Handful of fresh parsley

Add all ingredients except the mushrooms and parsley to the broth and gently simmer for 20 minutes. Add the sliced mushrooms and simmer for 10 more minutes. Remove the ginger and astragalus. Serve the soup in a bowl and top with raw parsley.

---

### BALSAM FIR (*Abies balsamea*)

Balsam fir is one of nine species of fir in North America. Its medicinal properties have long been recognized by indigenous peoples who use it widely. The resin is antiseptic and provides an analgesic, protective covering for burns, bruises, wounds, cuts, sprains, and sore nipples. The buds, resins, and sap have been used for cancer, corns, and warts. The Iroquois make a poultice of balsam fir gum mixed with dried beaver kidneys to treat cancer and also use a steam of the twigs during childbirth. An infusion of the leaves is used to treat cystitis, an infusion of the bark is used for tuberculosis, colds, and gonorrhea, and an infusion of the sap is used as an inhalant for headaches and is also an excellent remedy for a sore throat. Finally, a decoction of the branches is used as a soothing bath for muscle pain. To make a soaking bath, take 6 ounces of branches and simmer for 1 hour in 4 cups of water and then strain and add to a hot bath and soak for 20 minutes.

### BASIL, ITALIAN (*Ocimum basilicum*) *See* page 110.

### BILBERRY (*Vaccinium myrtillus*)

The leaves and berries of the bilberry shrub are both medicinal. The berries are rich in anthocyanin, the blue-purple pigment that is one of nature's most powerful antioxidants. The fruit of the bilberry is astringent and an effective remedy for diarrhea. It is used for constipation and vomiting. Daily use of the berries is an effective vasodilator (a blood vessel dilator) and use of the whole plant helps night blindness and retinopathy. The fruit is also used for urinary tract infections (UTIs) and as a topical antiseptic and anti-inflammatory.

Women have higher rates of cataracts than men. There are many approaches to preventing or slowing cataracts. Cataracts occur in large part as a result of a process of oxidative stress and glycation. Glycation occurs in response to high blood-glucose levels when proteins and tissues are damaged. The eye is especially vulnerable to glycation. Risk factors include high sugar levels, diabetes, ultraviolet (UV) exposure from the sun, and a history of smoking or excessive alcohol use.

Bilberries and their anthocyanin-rich sisters—blueberries, raspberries, and huckleberries—are potent antioxidants and eye medicines. There are many ways to ingest them. You can eat the berries themselves, fresh or frozen, or consume them in bilberry liqueurs, cordials, and jams. These are commonly made in Europe and are available for purchase in the United States, though one must be careful about added sugar since that is a major culprit in cataract development.

To slow or prevent cataracts and improve overall eye health, combine a daily dose of 100 to 200 milligrams of bilberry fruit extract (standardized to 36 percent total anthocyanins) with added carotenoids lutein and zeaxanthin. Eat a diet rich in lutein foods, such as eggs, cooked spinach, kiwi, zeaxanthin-rich spirulina, and dark leafy greens.

### BLACK CUMIN SEEDS (*Nigella sativa*) *See* page 112.

### BLACK HAW (*Viburnum prunifolium*)

Black haw is a deciduous shrub native to North America. It has long been used by native women of North America to reduce uterine cramping and to prevent miscarriage. Historically, it was forced on women who were enslaved to counteract herbal abortifacients and ensure they did not have miscarriages. The bark of black haw contains scopoletin, a coumarin that relaxes the uterus, and salicin, an anti-inflammatory and pain reliever. A decoction of the bark is used to ease morning sickness and speed recovery after childbirth. Its antispasmodic function also makes it useful for bile duct cramping in gallbladder pain and it is often mixed with cramp bark for this purpose. Take 400 milligrams of dried bark root in a capsule 3 times a day.

CAUTION: Black haw is also used to reduce blood pressure and thus may be contraindicated in women with low blood pressure.

### BLUEBERRY (*Vaccinium corymbosum*; *Vaccinium angustifolium*)

We eat the berries of this healing plant (whose genus also includes cranberries, bilberries, and huckleberries) as a delicious antioxidant, but we often forget about using the leaf. Yet, a half cup of a blueberry leaf infusion helps to sustain the effects of insulin injections in the treatment of diabetes and can counteract the "rusting" effects of high blood glucose on arterial health. To prepare an infusion, steep 1 ounce of dried blueberry leaves (or 3 ounces fresh) in 2 cups of just-boiled water for 10 minutes. Strain and drink.

### BORAGE (*Borago officinalis*)

Borage is an annual flowering herb native to Europe and naturalized in the United States. The oil from the seeds is very high (24 percent) in gamma linolenic acid (GLA), which makes it essential in the treatment of skin disorders, inflammatory illnesses such as arthritis, and autoimmune disease. It also promotes brain health and treats depression. As one of the several plant seed oils rich in GLA, it should be part of one's daily intake for good mood, reproductive health, and skin care. An early English saying is "Borage gives courage."

Small amounts of borage oil can be added to infant formula to provide essential fatty acids that promote development in preterm infants. The oil can also be used for adrenal fatigue and to increase urine flow, prevent lung inflammation, promote sweating, calm nerves, increase breast milk production, lower blood pressure, and treat bronchitis and colds. The flowers and leaves are used to treat fever, cough, and depression. The fresh leaves of the borage plant have a crisp, cucumber scent and are cooling additions to soups and salads.

### BOSWELLIA (*Boswellia serrata*)

Boswellia is also known as Indian frankincense, a tree native to India and used in Ayurvedic medicine. It is a potent anti-inflammatory and antiarthritic herb often used as part of herbal pain compounds. The resins are the medicinal part of the tree and are harvested by making incisions in the trees and collecting the gum. The two active compounds in boswellia are boswellin and boswellic acid. Boswellia is also beneficial for treating bronchial asthma and Crohn's disease, relieving menstrual cramps, and stimulating menstrual flow. It is a healthy and effective alternative to nonsteroidal anti-inflammatory drugs (NSAIDs).

The recommended dose is 300 to 600 milligrams 2 to 3 times a day. Use products with 40 to 60 percent boswellic acids.

### BUCHU (*Agathosma betulina*)

The shrubby buchu plant is native to western South Africa and a member of the lemon and orange family. The leaves of the plant are often combined with corn silk, juniper, and uva ursi to treat UTIs. A strong tea applied topically acts as an insect repellant. It is also a strong diuretic, so use with caution. Make a mild tea by steeping 1 gram of dried plant material in a cup of water for 15 minutes and drinking 2 cups a day for 2 days as a diuretic. Add 1 gram each of corn silk, juniper, uva ursi, and buchu to 1 quart of gently simmering water for 15 minutes and strain. Drink ½ cup 3 times a day for a UTI infection.

### BURDOCK (*Arctium lappa*)

Burdock is a detoxifying plant that nourishes the liver and kidneys. It is a potent blood tonic and it cleanses the skin and improves digestion by stimulating bile production. The roots and leaves are essential ingredients of culinary medicine. Burdock root shines when combined with other stimulating herbs like dandelion root for detoxification, and it is useful in treating UTIs. A decoction of the root or seed is a strong diuretic and a lymphatic cleanser and can be used to reduce swollen lymph nodes. It is a member of the daisy family, so if you allergic to daisies or ragweed you should avoid burdock.

→ *Bone Broth with Burdock* ←

Bone broth provides a perfect base for adding burdock root and dandelion root to one's diet. These herbs, like most roots, are best prepared in decoction. The following recipe is useful for recovery from chronic illness and acute virus infections.

**MAKES 12 SERVINGS**

1 ounce dandelion root

1 ounce burdock root

4 cloves garlic

4 thumbs fresh ginger

4 thumbs fresh turmeric

3 to 5 pounds marrowbones *or* chicken
    bones, including extra chicken feet for
    added collagen

1½ gallons water

3 teaspoons apple cider vinegar

A few handfuls fresh shiitake
    mushrooms, sliced

Put the dandelion root, burdock root, garlic, ginger, and turmeric inside a 4 inch by 4 inch square of double-thickness unbleached cheesecloth, fold all sides in, and tie with a cloth string. Set aside.

Put the bones in a large stock pot and pour over the water and apple cider vinegar. Let the bones rest for 1 hour. Bring the mixture to a boil over medium-high heat and then reduce to low heat and allow it to simmer for 8 to 12 hours. The longer your broth simmers, the better it gets. Add more water if necessary to make sure the bones are covered throughout the simmering process, until the final hour or so when the liquid may be allowed to reduce by half. Add the cheesecloth bundle or roots and herbs to your pot during the last 25 minutes of decoction. When finished, strain all solids from the broth using a fine mesh sieve. Add the shiitake mushrooms and allow them to soften in the hot broth. Let the decoction cool and then store in the refrigerator to enjoy throughout the week. Depending on the amount of time you allow the broth to simmer you will have about 12 to 16 cups of broth. Sip 1 cup of broth 3 times a day.

## CALENDULA (*Calendula officinalis*)

Calendula is the premier herb for skin salves and ointments used for eczema, hemorrhoids, chapped skin, diaper rash, minor cuts and burns, athlete's foot, acne, and varicose veins. An infusion of the flower can be used for swollen glands and inflammation of the mouth and throat. Calendula is combined with marshmallow root for stomach ulcers, with valerian or cramp bark for cramps, with peppermint for indigestion, and with blackberry root for diarrhea. It is also used in eardrop formulas that include mullein, yarrow, and garlic to treat ear infections in children. Grow calendula in a pot in a sunny window or in your garden and pick the flowers as you need. Infuse 4 flowers in a cup of boiled hot water and drink as a natural anti-inflammatory or to bring on menses. Dry extra flowers by placing them on paper for 1 week in a dark, dry place and store in a jar once fully dried. Homeopathic calendula spray is widely available for purchase for your first aid kit.

## → *Flower Petal Salad* ←

The edible flower heads of calendula are an effective treatment for anything related to the skin, and there are many additional flowers to add to your plate. Eating flower petals adds zest and pizazz to a salad. When you eat edible flowers make sure that they have not been sprayed.

Consider a lettuce and chickweed salad as the base and then add a light olive oil and citrus dressing. Make sure that you place the dressing at the bottom of the bowl, tossing the greens first and then add the flowers, as they will get drenched in the dressing and will lose their delicate shape and flavor.

**MY FAVORITE FLOWERS TO EAT**

Borage

Calendula

Clover

Dandelions

Nasturtiums (*Tropaeolum*)

Marigold (*Calendula officinalis*)

Pansies (*Viola tricolor*)

Roses (*Rosa*)

Squash blossoms (*Cucurbita pepo*)

---

**CANNABIS (*Cannabis sativa*) See page 133.**

**CAPOMO/BREADNUT/RAMON (*Brosimum alicastrum*)**
I set off one morning with my friend José Lorenzo Garcia to collect capomo. We walked for about thirty minutes before we reached an area of Jose's land, called Habita, high in the dry forest of Cabo Corrientes. There we found a tall capomo tree at the foot of a steep bank covered with a variety of veining flora. Around the base of the tree and beyond we collected the fallen capomo nuts or seeds, which are about the size of a round grape—some with green skin dotted with tiny bubbling dots and others a smooth brown, having been denuded by the bats the night before. The bats eat the thin-skinned fruit off the seed and then drop the seed for us to collect. While we were gathering, José explained that January through March is the best time to collect capomo. Some trees bear fruit every year; others biannually. Our four-footed animal friends—pigs, cows, and horses—also love capomo. Cows that are fed capomo leaves produce one to two liters more milk per day than cows fed on pasture, and pigs grow larger and healthier.

Capomo—also known as ramon or the breadnut—is a tasty coffee substitute, widespread on both coasts of Mexico. This nut has been an important traditional food and beverage commonly used by peoples throughout the east and west coasts of Mexico and in the jungles of Guatemala and is currently being revitalized as part of community healing strategies.

Capomo's special quality is that it provides significant levels of folate and all the essential amino acids. Capomo is a galactagogue used by new mothers, both human and swine. It is especially high in methionine, which helps the liver process fat and toxins, and tryptophan, an amino acid that is energizing and relaxing, as it lifts the mood. Capomo is also high in fiber, calcium, potassium, iron, zinc, protein, and vitamins A, B, C, and E. The seeds when roasted for coffee or boiled for bread have the protein equivalent of eggs. The flour is nutritionally superior and is ideal for people with gluten sensitivity. Capomo is now available in the United States (see "Resources" for a list of medicinal herb suppliers) and is also contained in the beverage Teeccino.

### → *Café de Capomo* ←

Prepare 2 tablespoons of ground capomo per cup of water in a French press or any other way that you would prepare coffee. Optionally add a pinch of cinnamon, nutmeg, vanilla, or chocolate to add aromatic flavor. You can also obtain capomo in a variety of commercial coffee substitutes. After you make the beverage, save the leftover grinds and add them to some capomo chocolate muffins!

**CARAWAY (*Carum carvi*) *See* page 113.**

**CARDAMOM (*Elettaria cardamomum*) *See* page 113.**

**CATNIP (*Nepeta cataria*)**
Cats love catnip, in part due to the nepetalactone it contains. This compound causes euphoria in most cats and mild sedation in humans. *Nepeta* derives from the Greek word *nēpenthés*, which refers to the drug of forgetfulness that was given to Helen of Troy in the *Odyssey*. Catnip is a member of the mint family and is rich in vitamins C and E. The infused tea helps as a febrifuge and diaphoretic and is used, along with bilberries, to prevent cataracts in humans. Pour a cup of hot water over 2 teaspoons of the dried flowers and leaves, then cover and let sit for 10 minutes before straining and drinking. Catnip stimulates menses and calms muscle spasms, and the juice of the fresh leaves can be applied to relieve hemorrhoids. Place an ounce each in a few bowls around the house (on a high shelf if you have children and animals) or near doorways, behind the fridge, or near trashcans to repel mosquitoes and cockroaches.

## CATTAILS (*Typha latifolia*)

Cattails are a genus of wetland species that have a wide range of ethnobotanical uses, from food to shelter, furniture, and clothing. The Snohomish people of the Pacific Northwest United States call cattail a "string made of leaf" since the fibrous leaves produce material for weaving mats, shades, clothing, and even fishing nets.

The starchy rhizome is edible and, along with the pollen, is ground and used as a flour substitute or added to food as a thickener. The leaves and pollen from the plant are diuretic. The dried pollen also has anticoagulant qualities and is used along with the ground root in the treatment of kidney stones, painful menstruation, abnormal uterine bleeding, and cystitis. Poultices from the bruised root are applied to cuts, wounds, burns, and stings. Cattail flowers are used to treat diarrhea and indigestion, and the ash of burned cattail leaves is antiseptic and styptic.

### ⇢ *Gathering and Making Cattail Flour* ⇠

Gather cattails during a wading adventure in the spring to collect their edible stalks and again later in the summer for their flowers and pollen. Cattail flour is made from the stalk. It should be cut just above the root and just before the green of the stalk. Bake the stalks in a 200°F oven for about 4 hours. Once they are dried out, pulverize them into flour. The flour will have fibers, or stringy parts, that don't break down when you pulverize the stalk. These should be removed before using the flour. You can add cattail flour to other nongluten flours and make treats like pancakes topped with blueberry sauce.

## CAYENNE (*Capsicum annuum*) *See* page 114.

## CHAI HU (*Bupleurum chinense*)

Chai hu is a member of the parsley family and native to central Asia. It is known as Free and Easy Wanderer because it helps move chi energy throughout the body and aids the process of "flow," of letting go and allowing for change. Chai hu protects the liver against stress. It aids in phase 2 liver detoxification and relief of PMS, depression, and vertigo. It can be added to a tea of ginger root, ginseng, and licorice root to support adrenal gland function when recovering from chronic stress and trauma.

*Bupleurum chinense* is part of a formula of seven herbs (bupleurum root, pinellia tuber, scutellaria root, jubube fruit, ginseng root, glycyrrhiza root, and ginger) used in Chinese Medicine called Xiao Chai Hu Tang used for treatment of liver damage and hepatitis C. Yet there are also reports of it causing hepatotoxicity in people with liver disease, suggesting that if you have liver disease, only use this formula under the guidance of an herbalist. The American species *Bupleurum americanum* is known as American thorowax and has similar properties, but it is more difficult to obtain. Like many herbs, it should be used for a specific purpose, short-term, and then rotated out while other herbs are used.

**CHAMOMILE (*Matricaria chamomilla*; *Chamaemelum nobile*) See page 116.**

**CHASTEBERRY, OR VITEX (*Vitex agnus-castus*)**
The berry of the chaste tree is used to stabilize and balance hormonal fluctuations especially related to progesterone. Chasteberry, or vitex, is useful in treating PMS and irregular menstruation, reducing menopausal symptoms, and stabilizing menses for those who are withdrawing from pharmaceutical birth control. It has also been used to help regulate ovulation for those trying to conceive. The name *vitex* is derived from the plant's anaphrodisiac qualities, though it has seemingly opposite effects for different people. For example it acts as both an aphrodisiac and an anaphrodisiac, reinforcing its role as bringer of the hormonal balance. The berry can be ingested as a tincture, decoction, syrup, or elixir, or eaten raw. Results are best achieved from long-term use. The exact mechanism by which vitex works is not well understood, but it is thought to normalize progesterone levels through the pituitary-hypothalamic axis, rather than stimulating the release of progesterone. To make the infusion, add 1 teaspoon of crushed berries to 1 cup of just-boiled water and steep, covered, for 10 to 15 minutes. Drink this infusion 3 times a day or take a tincture or capsule form (1,000 milligrams) in the morning.

**CHIA (*Salvia hispanica*)**
This superfood is also known as chian, chia sage, salba, and mila. It is one of the most important plant foods and medicines native to Mexico and served as one of four main foods, along with maize, frijoles, and amaranth, in pre-Spanish Mexico. *Chian* is a Nahuatl word meaning "by the water." The tiny mottled black and white seed cannot grow north of the twentieth parallel since it requires a natural altitude of between 1,500 and 5,000 feet above sea level.

Chia is a rich source of essential fatty acids, protein, antioxidants, and dietary fiber. Chia seed is 63 percent oil and the richest plant source of omega-3 fatty acids. The oil contains a perfect 1:2 ratio between omega-6 and omega-3 fatty acids. Eating chia during the final stages of pregnancy and early stages of breastfeeding results in higher levels of docosahexaenoic acid (DHA) in breastmilk. DHA is the essential fatty acid that is fundamental to brain, kidney, and eye development. Chia aids blood sugar metabolism, contributes to the relief of depression and anxiety, and reduces inflammation contributing to arthritis and cardiovascular disease. Chia seed is rich in iron and quercetin (a powerful antioxidant and anti-allergen).

Chia is also hydrophilic. It holds twelve times its weight in water. This "water clinging to seeds" results in body rehydration at the cellular level when you consume small quantities. These hydrophilic colloids also provide soothing action on intestinal walls, which makes chia a useful food when recovering from dysentery or illness. It also makes a valuable addition to fluid foods for elders or cancer patients who have lost their appetite. Chia enhances weight loss as it stimulates metabolism and reduces the appetite. It also lowers blood sugar and supports belly fat loss.

Chia is very versatile; put a tablespoon of the seeds in a glass with 8 ounces of water and let sit overnight in the fridge, squeeze in some fresh lemon juice, and drink it as a morning beverage. You may substitute coconut milk or cream for the water and add a few more tablespoons of the seeds to make a delicious chia coconut pudding topped with sliced banana. A tablespoon or two of dried chia is also a good addition to pancakes or muffins.

### CHICKWEED (*Stellaria media*)

While chickweed, a native of Europe, is often referred to as an invasive weed in North America, it is a wonderful herb to add to a fresh leaf salad. Chickweed has anti-inflammatory and nourishing qualities. It is also used externally as a demulcent and emollient for rashes, eczema, stings, and diaper rash. The boiled leaves of chickweed taste like spring spinach. The fresh aerial parts of the plant can be preserved in alcohol as a tincture, which can be used for interstitial cystitis and ovarian cysts. A very simple tincture is to fill a jar ¾ of the way with fresh chickweed and cover with vodka. Tightly screw on a lid and let it sit in a dark shelf for 4 weeks, shaking daily. Take 15 drops 3 times a day. Chickweed is one of seven herbs used in a traditional Japanese dish served during *Nanakusa no sekku*, the "Festival of Seven Herbs," which celebrates longevity.

### CILANTRO, CORIANDER (*Coriandrum sativum*) *See* page 117.

## CLEAVERS (*Galium aparine*)

Cleavers is an annual, herbaceous plant in the coffee family. The name derives from the way the plant shoots cling to anything they touch with tiny little hooks. An ancient medicinal plant, cleavers is used for all things urinary: UTIs, kidney stones, inflammation, and acidic urine. The Ojibway use the plant as a diuretic. The fruit of the plant can be dried, roasted, and used as a coffee substitute, and the tips of the young plants are eaten raw in salads. Cleavers can be used as a tea, or the plant can be juiced and preserved with vegetable glycerin and used as a cleansing spring tonic for the lymphatic system and liver. Take 10 grams of fresh leaves and steep in hot water, strain, and drink 3 times daily for 7 days for acute care. The asperuloside in cleavers functions as a mild laxative, and the Cherokee use an infusion of it for just that purpose. The Ojibway use a cold infusion topically for poison ivy. Dried cleavers is also used to stuff mattresses.

## COFFEE (*Coffea arabica*) *See* page 135.

## COHOSH, BLACK (*Actaea racemosa*)

Black cohosh is a member of the buttercup family and is native to North America. Its root is used to help bring balance to the female reproductive system at all stages of life. It helps painful and delayed menstruation and is used to aid in childbirth by stimulating intermittent contractions of the uterus. It also helps menopause-related vasomotor symptoms, such as hot flashes. The root of black cohosh is a popular nervine, beneficial for treating numbness, neuralgia, and insomnia. For insomnia and anxiety make a tea combining black cohosh root, skullcap, wood betony (*Stachys officinalis*), passionflower, and valerian root.

Recommended dose and preparations include a decoction made by adding 1 teaspoon of the root to 1 cup water and simmering, covered, for 10 to 15 minutes. It can be sweetened with stevia if desired and drunk up to 3 times a day. A commercial standardized product called Remifemin is also available. Take 20 milligrams 2 to 3 times a day. Current evidence does not suggest that black cohosh is associated with an increased risk of breast cancer.

## COHOSH, BLUE (*Caulophyllum thalictroides*)

Blue cohosh has long been used for the induction of childbirth. Used traditionally by Native American women to aid in labor, blue cohosh became popular among allopathic physicians and midwives in the United States during the nineteenth century and remained a part of its official pharmacopoeia until 1890. Despite this history, most herbalists have now agreed to stop using blue cohosh during all stages of pregnancy because of concerns about its safety and efficacy. However, it is still used by many midwives during labor. Its historical use as an abortifacient, which is in keeping with its ability to induce labor, makes blue cohosh especially inappropriate in earlier stages of pregnancy. It is thought that the same saponin constituents that are responsible for its uterine stimulant effects are also likely to be toxic to the heart. Studies also suggest that blue cohosh may damage mitochondrial function. All of these studies have led to a reevaluation of blue cohosh and have concluded that it should not be recommended as safe to use during pregnancy or labor.

### COPAIBA (*Copaifera langsdorffii*)

Copaiba balsam is a natural oleoresin derived from the trunks of a variety of trees from the *Copaifera* genus found in South America. Indigenous peoples of the Americas have commonly used the oil for healing. It is possible that observing animals rubbing themselves on the copaiba tree trunks to heal their wounds proved instructive. It is anti-inflammatory and used topically for pain, bruises, and fungal infections. It is advisable to test a drop or two on a small skin area to determine your sensitivity.

CAUTION: Copaiba should not be taken internally.

### CORN SILK (*Zea mays*)

Associated with the mother goddess in Mexico for more than 6,000 years and in North America for about 1000 years, corn provides her long silky threads for our health. These stringy tassels are effective in treating urinary infections and kidney stones and are potent diuretics, reducing edema in diabetes. The silk contains saponin and allantoin compounds and is a potent antioxidant. When buying corn, make sure you buy non-genetically modified organism (non-GMO) varieties. Collect the silk during the summer when corn is fresh, tie the ends together, and then hang them up in a cool dry place until dry. Store for later use. Make an infusion by adding a handful of dried or fresh silk to a cup of hot water. Let it steep for 20 minutes and drink 3 cups a day. Alternatively take a tincture, 5 to 15 milliliters (1:5 at 25%), up to 3 times a day. Corn silk is very safe.

### CORYDALIS (*Corydalis yanhusuo*; *Corydalis cava*)

Related to the flowering poppy, the corydalis is often used as an analgesic and an alterative. In Chinese Medicine it is regarded as "invigorating" to the blood and traditionally has been used for menstrual cramps and abdominal pains and to strengthen circulation. The species *Corydalis cava* has been used to treat Parkinson's disease and other neurological disorders. The root of the plant is dried and made into a decoction or tincture. These are both potent plants and should be used under the guidance of a professional.

### CRAMP BARK (*Viburnum opulus*)

As the name implies, cramp bark is an effective uterine antispasmodic, making it very useful for treating menstrual cramps and regulating menstruation. The bark can be made into a decoction or tincture and can be used for acute uterine problems or as a general uterine tonic. Take 2 teaspoons of dried bark and simmer in 2 cups of water for 15 minutes and drink 1 to 2 cups a day as needed. For a tincture use 4 to 10 milliliters (1:5 at 45%) up to 3 times a day during menses. The active components of cramp bark are hydroquinones, arbutins, and coumarins along with astringent tannins.

### CRANBERRY (*Vaccinium Oxycoccos*; *Vaccinium macrocarpon*)

A cranberry is the tart fruit of an evergreen, dwarf shrub. The fruit is frequently made into a juice or sauce and is high in arbutin, a compound that fights infection and prevents bacteria, including E. coli, from clinging to the bladder. Indigenous peoples of North America use cranberry generously in their diets. Cranberry juice is a diuretic and also helps to alleviate symptoms of UTIs. You can take it in capsule form, 400 to 1,000 milligrams daily for a UTI, or extracts standardized to 25 percent proanthocyanidins 3 to 4 times a day.

### CULVER'S ROOT (*Veronicastrum virginicum*)

Culver's root is an herbaceous perennial, native to North America, and widely used among indigenous peoples as a detoxifying blood cleanser and a purgative and to stimulate the liver and bile flow. The root is also used as a diaphoretic and a disinfectant and to alleviate back pain. An infusion of the dried roots makes a strong laxative. The dried roots are milder and are best if dried for at least a year in a dark, cool place before use. Take 1 milliliter of extract (1:3 at 65%) up to twice daily.

### DAMIANA (*Turnera diffusa*; *Turnera*)

A small, woody shrub with aromatic flowers that grows in hot, humid climates, damiana is most notably used as an aphrodisiac and anxiety reducer. It is also an antispasmodic and helps reduce menstrual pain and blood sugar in diabetes. The dried leaves and twigs can be used as a tincture or tea, and they are often combined with ginseng or maca. The leaves can also be smoked. See pages 248–49 for several recipes for damiana, including a liqueur.

### DANDELION (*Taraxacum campylodes*)

If you are lucky enough to have dandelions in your yard, pluck them out of the ground when they are fresh. The leaves, root, and pretty yellow flowers can be used medicinally in many ways, including in dandelion wine.

There are many ways to benefit from dandelions. While they are both a bitter and a tonic, their fresh leaves added to salad perk up an otherwise less interesting dish. They can also be steamed and topped with butter as the fat in the butter will aid absorption of vitamin A and also stimulate the liver. Boiling the root makes a fine after-meal tea.

Though the whole plant can be used, the roots are the most medicinally potent. The leaves have diuretic qualities and a high mineral content. The plant contains bitter principles, making it helpful for stimulating the secretion of bile and removing excess water from the body. Dandelion can be taken in a variety of ways, fresh or dried. Roasted dandelion root can be drunk as a coffee substitute, often mixed with other roasted plants. Dandelion is mild and safe and an important herb to take as a part of a balanced, nutritious diet.

### DEVIL'S CLAW (*Harpagophytum procumbens*)

The name *devil's claw* means "hook plant" in Greek, and it is a powerful analgesic and anti-inflammatory. Take a tincture 3 times daily between meals for 2 to 3 months.

### DONG QUAI (*Angelica sinensis*)

Called the Empress of Herbs, dong quai is one of the most important herbs and spices in Chinese Medicine for women's health. It is a foundational herb for regulating the menstrual cycle and reducing menopausal symptoms such as hot flashes.

It is considered estrogenic because of its use as a female tonic herb, yet its exact mechanism of action is not well understood. Dong quai has a long history of being used to balance and normalize hormone production and reduce fatigue. Rosemary Gladstar suggests that it strengthens and tonifies the uterus. It is a mild, relaxing nervine and nourishing to the blood, so it is beneficial for delayed menstruation or for women with menopausal symptoms. It may also be useful in preventing osteoporosis and rheumatoid arthritis. Dong quai is often used as a spice in soups. The root can be prepared in capsule or tincture form, or dried root slices can be used in a decoction. The recommended dose ranges from 2 to 3 grams of root a day.

CAUTION: Dong quai should not be used while actively menstruating or during pregnancy.

### ECHINACEA (*Echinacea*; *Echinacea purpurea*; *Echinacea angustifolia*)

Echinacea is one the most popular immune system–enhancing herbs. It is useful for any respiratory condition, including strep throat, bronchitis, asthma, sinusitis, cough, or head colds. Applied topically, it reduces skin inflammation and joint pain and soothes sunburn. The dose used depends upon the part of the plant used and the duration of use. Treatment for an acute infection (colds, herpes, etc.) can be dosed at 0.9 milliliter, 5 to 6 times a day for up to 1 week, and for daily preventative use for an infection, take it 3 times per day for up to 4 weeks.

CAUTION: Echinacea stimulates phagocytosis (a process that awakens the immune system) and it is a matter of controversy whether it is contraindicated in people who have autoimmune disorders.

### ELDERFLOWER (*Sambucus*; *Sambucus nigra*)

Elderflower, or elderberry, also referred to as black elderberry, is a large shrub, all of which provides medicine. The bark is a strong purgative, an ointment made of the leaves acts as an emollient and is helpful for bruises, an infusion of the flowers will bring on a strong sweat, due to their rich flavonoid and phenolic compounds, and the berries have powerful antiviral and immune enhancing properties. The elderflower plant and berries are poisonous in their natural form, so they need to be heated and processed to remove the toxic cyanogenic glycosides (similar to apple seeds). The flowers and berries are traditionally made into syrup or extract and used for flus, colds, sore throats, and bronchitis. A poultice made from the flowers reduces swelling.

### ELECAMPANE (*Inula helenium*)

The roots of the elecampane plant might be your first choice for treating bronchial congestion, asthma, and chronic cough and to aide menstrual flow. It contains inulin, which acts as an expectorant, toning and clearing the pulmonary membranes. As a prebiotic, inulin helps feed healthy gut bacteria and relieve an upset stomach. The elecampane root has long been sacred to Celtic peoples. It is bitter and not very palatable, but you can add lemon and honey to a decoction or use an extract or glycerite made from the fresh root. The sesquiterpene lactones in the plant are antibacterial.

---

⇉ *Candied Elecampane Lozenges* ⇇

Elecampane makes an effective candied lozenge for coughs and excess mucus. It is also good for providing an energy boost during recovery after a long illness. One can use a variety of sugars (raw honey, coconut sugar), but I like to use dark agave syrup that is rich in minerals and matches well with the bitterness of this healing root.

Take 4 ounces of fresh cleaned root and 4 ounces of dark agave syrup. The roots should be cut into bite-size pieces that you will suck and chew. Put the syrup in a small pan and heat on low and as it warms and thins, add the roots. You might want to add a few tablespoons of water if the agave is very thick. Be sure the roots are fully covered by the syrup. Bring the mixture to a light boil and cook until clumps start to form. Pour onto wax paper or unbleached parchment paper, separate out the root pieces, and let them dry. If you live in a moist climate you might need to freeze them briefly. Store in a large, dry amber glass bottle.

---

### ELEUTHERO, A.K.A. SIBERIAN GINSENG (*Eleutherococcus senticosus*)

Eleuthero, also known as Siberian ginseng, is a small shrub native to Asia. The roots of the plant are adaptogenic and stimulating. They are used to treat fatigue, lack of concentration, or exhaustion due to overwork. Their active constituents include eleutherosides and complex polysaccharides, which are responsible for supporting immune function and increasing stamina and endurance. The plant also stimulates T-cell production, helps to maintain good health, and improves the capacity for exercise by enhancing oxygen uptake. The standard dose ranges from 1,200 to 1,600 milligrams daily in capsules or extract. There are no serious adverse effects related to the use of eleuthero, though excessive use may induce euphoria and insomnia.

### EVENING PRIMROSE (*Oenothera*; *Oenothera biennis*)

Originating in North America the oil in the seeds of the evening primrose are rich in GLA, making it essential in the treatment of dermatological health, especially atopic eczema and acne. It is also used to treat PMS, menopause symptoms, and rheumatoid arthritis. The standard dose is 1,000 to 2,000 milligrams of oil daily.

### EYEBRIGHT (*Euphrasia*)

As its name implies, eyebright is a traditional remedy for any ailment affecting the eyes—conjunctivitis, allergy-related weeping, sties, and poor vision. It is helpful in treating dry eye, which can occur with age. The iridoid glycosides in eyebright decrease swelling and are antibacterial and antifungal. Eyebright is also used for respiratory ailments and sinus congestion due to allergies. Eyebright makes an excellent eyewash, eyedrop, and eye compress. A tincture of eyebright can also be taken internally to enhance eyesight.

### → *Eyebright Eyewash* ←

The key to making an effective eyewash is to ensure that all materials are sterilized and clean and no bits of plant material get into the eye. There are many fine washes on the market as well. Bring 2 cups of water to a boil and pour over 4 tea bags of eyebright or ½ ounce of the leaf. Steep for 20 minutes. Strain the liquid through very fine cheesecloth twice, let cool, and add to a sterile bottle with eyedropper. You can use a dropper to drop 6 drops into the corner of each eye or use an eyewash cup. Store in the fridge for up to 1 week. Before use, let it return to room temperature. Use 3 times a day for 3 days for acute inflammation or irritation, or daily to improve sight or to address dry eye or irritation.

### FENNEL (*Foeniculum vulgare*) *See* page 122.

### FENUGREEK (*Trigonella foenum-graecum*)

Fenugreek seeds are native to Asia and southern Europe. They are rich in soluble fiber, which helps to lower blood sugar by slowing the absorption of carbohydrates. Fenugreek soothes digestion, reduces gas, relieves allergies, and loosens mucus. The seeds have a small amount of the amino acid L-tryptophan and contain natural phytoestrogens, such as diosgenin, making it helpful for menopause symptoms and painful menstruation. It is also a galactagogue, so it increases breast milk. In addition, fenugreek reduces pain, boosts the immune system, reduces cholesterol levels, and relieves constipation. Sprout the seeds or take a tablespoon of the seeds and simmer them in 2 cups of water for 15 minutes, strain, and drink.

### FEVERFEW (*Tanacetum parthenium*)

Also known as Santa Maria and bachelor's button, these flowers look similar to the chamomile flower. Feverfew is my go-to herb for the treatment of headaches, specifically migraines. It was considered the "aspirin" of the seventeenth century. It is also an effective febrifuge, as its name suggests. It is analgesic, anti-inflammatory, and antispasmodic. It also inhibits serotonin binding, which is a central factor of migraines, and decreases the intensity of symptoms associated with migraine, including nausea, visual auras, vomiting, and light and smell sensitivity. It also has uterine-stimulating effects, which aligns with its use in traditional medicine as both an abortifacient and emmenagogue. The tea is also used as an anxiolytic and antidepressant.

To treat a migraine or fever, steep 3 fresh leaves and drink as a tea twice a day or take 400 to 1,200 milligrams over the course of a day in 4 divided doses standardized to contain 0.2 to 0.4 percent parthenolides.

CAUTION: Fresh feverfew leaves can cause contact dermatitis in some people.

### FIGS AND FIG LEAVES (*Ficus carica*)

The fig tree, a member of the mulberry family, has figured prominently in the world's religions. Muslims called the fig the Tree of Heaven, Adam and Eve in the Judeo-Christian Bible wrapped themselves in fig leaves, and Buddha sat under the bodhi tree, the sacred fig (*ficus religiosa*), until he gained enlightenment.

The fruit of the fig tree is rich in calcium and iron, making it a useful food for anemia. Figs are also antispasmodic, effective as a mild laxative, and useful as an emollient for intestinal griping. Split a fresh fig in half and apply it to a boil to soften it before applying heat to drain the boil. Fresh figs may be roasted and applied warm to gum inflammation, and fig leaves are hypoglycemic and can be cooked and stuffed with food.

### FLAX (*Linum usitatissimum*)

Flaxseeds are rich in proteins, lignans, and omega-3 fatty acids. Consuming flaxseed every day reduces the intensity of hot flashes during menopause. Flaxseed also helps in reducing bone loss, stabilizing blood sugar, lowering cholesterol, promoting weight loss, and boosting immunity. People with autoimmune and inflammatory disorders can benefit from a regular consumption of flax. Flaxseed oil can be added to salad dressing, and ground flaxseed makes an excellent base for an herbal poultice.

## FUNGI

Fungi are eukaryotic organisms and include mushrooms and microorganisms such as yeasts and molds. They are not herbs per se, but they form an important part of our natural repertoire for healing and are often used with herbal medicines. Many mushrooms contain extraordinary health properties—they are antioxidant, anti-inflammatory, antiviral, antimicrobial, antihypertensive, and immune enhancing. Medicinal fungi have complex carbohydrates called polysaccharides, which are responsible for stimulating and enhancing the immune system and may explain the purported anticancer properties of fungi.

Mushrooms are easy to assimilate into a diet since they can function both as food and medicine. Besides having a strong influence on the immune system when needed, fungi can be used as preventative medicine and as adaptogens. Some common health concerns fungi can remedy include sleep disturbances, seasonal allergies, the common cold, weak hair and skin, low athletic performance, low sex drive, low energy, high stress and cortisol production, liver congestion, high cholesterol, high blood sugar, weight issues, digestive complaints, joint pain, mood disturbances, and poor concentration. See chapter 6 for a discussion of a few psychoactive plants and mushrooms.

The fungi I invite you to explore for your diet include lion's mane (*Hericium erinaceus*), shiitake (*Lentinula edodes*), cordyceps, reishi, maitake (*Grifola frondosa*), chaga (*Inonotus obliquus*), turkey tail or cloud mushroom (*Trametes versicolor*), and mesima (*Phellinus linteus*). Freshly gathered fungi may be found in local farmers markets or grocery stores. The dosing of medicinal mushrooms depends upon the strength of the extract and you will want to explore the reliable suppliers of medicinal grade mushroom extracts (see "Resources").

## GARLIC (*Allium sativum*)

Garlic is the essential heal-all. Before penicillin was identified, garlic was the herbal antibiotic of choice and also functioned as a powerful antifungal; garlic suppositories are effective treatments for yeast infections. Garlic has immune-enhancing effects and should be part of a regular diet to decrease the occurrences of colds, flu, and bronchitis. It lowers high blood pressure and cholesterol and is helpful with E. coli and salmonella infections. Garlic is rich in the sulfur that supports phase 2 liver detoxification and is also part of an overall repertoire to lift depression.

## ⇾ *Simple Garlic Onion Soup* ⇽

There are so many wonderful ways to benefit from garlic: eating it raw in salad dressings, adding it to soups and vegetables, slow baking whole garlic heads. There is even garlic ice cream!

I love making this garlic onion soup at least every few weeks. It's rich and warming, boosts immune function, and cleanses the liver and bloodstream. Concerned about garlic breath? Just chew on some fresh parsley and share your soup with everyone around you.

**SERVES 4**

4 whole garlic cloves

Virgin cold-pressed olive oil

2 large onions, thinly sliced

4 cups fresh chicken, beef, or
   vegetable broth

¼ cup white wine

Sea salt

Freshly cracked black pepper

¼ cup fresh parsley

Croutons (optional)

Hard goat cheddar (optional)

Cut the tops off the garlic heads just enough to expose the upper part of the clove. Drizzle olive oil over the heads, place them on a cookie sheet or small enamel dish, and bake them in the oven for 1 hour at 300°F. While the garlic is baking, put the onions in a large sauté pan with a little olive oil over low heat. Let them caramelize, stirring occasionally. When the onions are caramelized, turn off the heat and add the broth. When the garlic has finished baking, gently squeeze the cloves out of their skins and add them to the soup along with the white wine. Simmer the soup gently for 30 minutes so the flavors blend. Add salt and pepper to taste and serve, sprinkling some fresh parsley on top. As an option, you can also pour the soup into bowls prepared with croutons and hard goat cheddar.

---

### GINKGO (*Ginkgo biloba*)

The *Ginkgo biloba* tree is known as the maidenhair tree. It is the only living relative of the *Ginkgo* genus. Known as one of the oldest trees in the world, it has been found in fossils that are 270 million years old. It's immune to bugs and insects, fungi, and diseases. The ginkgo tree is among several trees that are called "survivor trees" because they survived the atomic blast in Hiroshima. Ginkgo has been used in Chinese Medicine for at least 5,000 years; the stinky fruit is used for asthma, allergies, and bronchitis. The leaves are used to improve brain function by increasing cerebral blood flow and protecting the brain from oxidative damage. The leaf extract or capsules are also used to treat anxiety, depression, memory impairment, poor concentration, vertigo, tinnitus, and macular degeneration. Its active constituents are ginkgo flavone glycosides and terpene lactones. A concentrated extract of 24 percent ginkgo flavone glycoside is the dose taken 3 times daily for at least 3 months for noticeable improvements in brain function. In my clinical experience some people can get headaches when using ginkgo. This could be due to the vasodilation effect, but if it persists, other herbs should be substituted.

### GINSENG, AMERICAN (*Panax quinquefolius*)
With many similar qualities to Korean, or Asian, ginseng (see below), American ginseng is called the "five fingers root." This variety of ginseng is on the endangered list in many states due to overharvesting. American ginseng is a member of the ivy family and improves cognitive function and memory. Three grams a day is safe for use in people with type 2 diabetes to prevent sharp rises in blood sugar, post meals. It is widely revered by indigenous peoples of North America who use it to aid recovery from illness and support reproductive well-being. American ginseng is used by women of the Meskwaki (Red Earth People) Nation as a love medicine to attract a partner. To enhance working memory and attention, take a ginseng product that has 5 to 50 milligrams of total ginsenosides. A standardized product called Cereboost is added to many herbal medicine products to support cognitive function.

### GINSENG, KOREAN (*Panax ginseng*)
The genus *Panax* is derived from the word *panacea*, meaning "heal-all." Ginseng is used as an adaptogen and an immunomodulator and thus is helpful when recovering from chronic illness and the effects of trauma and substance abuse. It supports the nervous system, dispels mental exhaustion, boosts the libido, eases menopausal transition, improves overall stamina, and increases resistance to disease. Korean ginseng (*Panax ginseng*), although similar to Siberian ginseng, is from an entirely different family. The root (in both the American and Asian variety) contains a group of ginsenosides, which contribute to increased energy, enhanced physical and mental performance, and regulation of a proper stress response. A standardized extract that contains 4 to 7 percent ginsenosides (100 to 200 milligrams) can be taken daily for 3 weeks. Then rest from the herb for 1 week before beginning again. A tea can also be made with the thoroughly dried root.

### GOLDENSEAL (*Hydrastis canadensis*)

The root of goldenseal contains high levels of hydrastine and berberine, making it a powerful herb to treat bacterial and fungal infections, especially candida overgrowth and small intestinal bacterial overgrowth. It is also an effective digestive stimulant, astringent, and anti-inflammatory. Consuming goldenseal stimulates the secretion of bile and nourishes mucous membranes. It is a bitter and astringent herb. Ingesting the whole plant is more effective than consuming the isolated alkaloid berberine, though berberine alone has been shown to be very effective in lowering blood sugar in type 2 diabetes. Due to overharvesting and habitat destruction, goldenseal is considered an endangered species. Use only cultivated goldenseal, in order to safeguard it in the wild. Goldenseal can be used in moderation when needed but not as a daily foundation herb. Oregon grape root, also rich in berberine, is an effective substitute for goldenseal. A capsule of 50 to 150 milligrams twice a day is an adequate dose for short-term treatment. Goldenseal interacts with the P450 enzyme in the liver so make sure that you explore potential interactions with other medications you are taking.

### GOTU KOLA, PENNYWORT (*Centella asiatica*)

Gotu kola is also known as pennywort and is one of the most important plants in Ayurvedic medicine, where it is considered one of the elixirs of life and called brahmi, the herb of enlightenment. Elephants are widely observed to eat its fresh leaves. It is effective in reducing stress and depression and strengthening adrenal glands. It is a brain and body restorative, a skin and tissue regenerator, and a nervine used to increase mental concentration and relaxation. Gotu kola has been shown to reduce the startle response in people with post-traumatic stress disorder (PTSD). It can be applied topically as an oil for healing wounds, though some people can be sensitive to it, and contains saponins, which aid in collagen production. Take either an extract or an infusion made from 1 to 2 teaspoons of the dried leaf in a cup of water taken 3 times a day.

### GYMNEMA (*Gymnema sylvestre*)

Gymnema is an important herb used for the prevention and management of type 2 diabetes and also for weight loss. The leaves of this herb suppress sugar cravings. The gymnemic acid molecules mimic the structure of the glucose molecules that trick the body into acting to reduce sugar cravings, therefore reducing blood sugar. Traditionally used in Ayurveda and widely used in Mexico, chewing or brewing gymnema leaves into a tea reduces blood glucose and decreases sugar consumption.

Gymnema leaves are also antimicrobial and hepatoprotective. Gymnema is an effective diuretic, laxative, and cough suppressant. Capsules should have at least 25 percent gymnemic acid and be taken 5 to 10 minutes before a meal.

### HAWTHORN LEAF AND BERRY (*Crataegus*)

There are about sixty species in the genus *Crataegus*, and the leaf, flower, and berry are perhaps the most important herbs for heart health. Anyone who is concerned about their heart function should incorporate hawthorn into their daily health routine. The fruits are rich in bioflavonoids with antioxidant effects and are often made into a jelly or wine. The leaves can be eaten in salads. An extract of hawthorn is effective in treating high or low blood pressure, strengthening the heart, normalizing heart rhythm, lowering high cholesterol, and decreasing fatty plaques in blood vessels. Hawthorn may also be useful for grief and sadness associated with loss, as it was known in ancient Europe as the "tree of love."

For heart conditions use a standardized extract and combine it with night-blooming cactus and motherwort. Make teas and syrups from the fruits, flowers, and berries, all of which are rich in antioxidants. Hawthorn also supports nitric oxide production, and a proprietary blend that includes beet extract is incorporated into sublingual tablets to restore nitric oxide function for arterial dilation and healthy blood flow. Take 500 milligram capsules 2 to 3 times a day.

### HOLY BASIL (Tulsi) (*Ocimum tenuiflorum*)

Holy basil is a sacred plant among the Hindu, and in Ayurvedic medicine it is known as the Mother Medicine of Nature revered for its spiritual and medicinal qualities. Named after Tulsi, the goddess of good fortune, it brings health through its adaptogenic qualities and treats a wide variety of health conditions, including metabolic syndrome (prediabetes). In traditional medicine it is an antifertility and abortifacient herb (possibly due to its testosterone-enhancing qualities). In addition to enhancing skin quality and protecting against environmental toxins, it reduces anxiety, depression, and stress and is a potent anti-inflammatory, antioxidant, and immunomodulator and it is also hepatoprotective and cardioprotective. It combines well with milk thistle when used to enhance liver health, and when used topically it has mosquito-repelling properties.

Traditionally, powdered tulsi is added to ghee and can be used during a meal. Make a cup of tea daily by adding 1 to 2 tablespoons to a cup of hot water to reduce stress and enhance well-being and save some to use as a cooling antibacterial mouthwash. Take 500 milligrams 2 to 3 times a day on an empty stomach, every day for 1 to 3 months.

CAUTION: The antifertility and abortifacient qualities of this plant suggest that it should not be used when trying to conceive or when pregnant.

### HONEYSUCKLE (*Lonicera periclymenum*)

Honeysuckle is one of the most important herbs used in Chinese Medicine. This plant climbs and clings and is thus called a love-binding plant that enhances fidelity in relationships. Honeysuckle flowers help to reduce hot flashes and fevers, suppress flus and other viruses, and reduce inflammatory processes in the body. It is used with chrysanthemum to lower high blood pressure. The crushed flowers rubbed on the third eye (the area located on the forehead between the eyebrows) are thought to enhance psychic vision. Make a tea from fresh flowers or obtain an essential oil, which has a light sweet smell, and use it with a diffuser for aromatherapy or to add to your shower or bath steam to induce relaxation.

### HOPS (*Humulus lupulus*)

The hops flower is used in beer making to add bitter, zesty flavors to the medicinal and sedative qualities of the brew. Hops is beneficial for treating anxiety, lack of appetite, and insomnia. It possesses potent estrogenic activity when fresh (which may account for the beer belly that male beer drinkers have). The strobiles (the cone-like parts of the plant) are made up of overlapping bracts and are useful in helping to delay menstruation. They are naturally very bitter, making the plant valuable in the treatment of digestive complaints, such as enhancing digestion by increasing gastric juices.

I combine hops with valerian and passionflower to synergize its effects, and it is commonly found in pill form in this combination. The recommended dose for hops alone is 300 to 500 milligrams before bed, as needed for relaxation and sleep.

### HORSETAIL (*Equisetum*)

Horsetail, called *cola de caballo* in Spanish, is an ancient plant that has grown from the earth for over 300 million years. The fresh shoots that rise in early spring are edible. Horsetail is an excellent diuretic, making it useful in reducing edema and in aiding urinary flow to reduce bacterial infections and inflammation of the lower urinary tract. It is rich in silica and other minerals, which makes it ideal for preventing and treating osteoporosis and enhancing hair and nail growth during menopause. Horsetail can staunch bleeding and heal wounds, ulcers, and skin inflammations when applied externally. To make a tea, grab a large handful of dried horsetail and simmer it in a quart of water for 20 minutes. Strain and pour a cup, adding a few sprigs of your favorite fresh mint to make a subtle tasting, medicinal beverage. Horsetail is fun to work with because it is made up of tough hollow stems that can be tied together and used to scrub your pots and pans while camping.

### HYSSOP (*Hyssopus officinalis*)

Hyssop is an effective cough expectorant and digestive aid. It is used in children and adults alike for common colds, bronchitis, asthma, and anxiety, and it functions as a peripheral vasodilator, diaphoretic, and anti-inflammatory. Inhaling hyssop vapors is an effective treatment option for upper respiratory conditions and tinnitus. While it is a mint, it can benefit from some honey or can be used in an extract. Hyssop can be taken as a tincture, a tea, or even made into an oxymel. Because hyssop is often made to address a cough or illness of a few days' duration, make enough for a few days by adding 1 cup of hyssop to a quart jar of boiled water. Cover the jar and let it sit overnight, straining the next day and adding a little raw local honey.

CAUTION: Hyssop is an emmenagogue and should not be used during pregnancy.

### JAMAICAN DOGWOOD (*Piscidia piscipula*)

Native to the Western Hemisphere, Jamaican dogwood root bark (the outer bark of the root) is an antispasmodic and analgesic and is useful for easing menstrual cramps. It is also useful as a sedative and, as such, is one of a number of plants that indigenous peoples traditionally place in a fishing area to sedate fish, so they are easier to catch. When using Jamaican dogwood obtain a professionally made tincture to ensure standardized quality and take 10 drops, 2 to 4 times a day between meals.

CAUTION: Some safety concerns suggest that this plant should only be used under the guidance of a professional. It should not be used on children or during pregnancy.

### JUNIPER BERRIES (*Juniperus*; *Juniperus communis*)

Juniper berries are used medicinally in the treatment of urinary complaints due to their mild diuretic and astringent qualities. The berries' volatile oil, terpinen-4-ol, increases the rate of kidney filtration, causing an increase in urine flow and removing waste and acidic toxins from the body. Their detoxifying qualities make the berries helpful in the treatment of inflammatory diseases like gout, rheumatoid arthritis, and bacterial and yeast infections. Commission E approves the use of juniper berries for indigestion, and they are often found in kidney-cleanse formulas. Juniper berries are also used to clear bronchial congestion and are antimicrobial, antifungal, and antiseptic. The oil of juniper berries applied topically is warming and stimulating. Indigenous peoples of the Pacific Northwest crush the berries to flavor deer meat. Make a gentle tea by crushing a tablespoon of berries and letting it steep in a cup of hot water. Keep the berries away from children and dogs as they can cause vomiting if eaten in large amounts.

### KUDZU (*Pueraria lobata*)

Often regarded as an invasive plant, kudzu is a member of the pea family, native to China where it's used in traditional medicine as a muscle relaxant and to treat high blood pressure and angina. Kudzu flowers and roots suppress alcohol cravings and enhance glutathione, a potent antioxidant that aids liver detoxification. Up to 2 to 3 grams of kudzu root extract daily can be used to decrease alcohol cravings.

### LADY'S MANTLE (*Alchemilla xanthochlora*)

Lady's mantle is a foundational herb for women's health used in the treatment of excessive menstruation and vaginitis. It is considered a magical plant as its name, *Alchemilla*, meaning "little alchemist," suggests. Stories from the Middle Ages tell that the dew that collects in her leaves is the purest source of water and was used in alchemical formulations. Lady's mantle is an astringent, tonic, diuretic, and anti-inflammatory. A freshly crushed poultice of leaves can be applied to cuts and wounds. Rich in tannins, it may be used in the treatment of diarrhea.

### LAVENDER (*Lavandula angustifolia*)

Lavender is one of the preeminent herbal sedatives that has both internal and external application. The inhaled oil used as aromatherapy is effective in the treatment of anxiety, depression, and pain. Internally, lavender is used for insomnia, IBS, flatulence, and stomach pain. Lavender reduces autonomic hyperarousal, suggesting its benefit in the treatment of trauma. Lavela WS 1265 is a patented formula of lavender essential oil that has been well studied for internal use for the treatment of anxiety, restlessness, and insomnia. The recommended dose is 80 to 160 milligrams per day for adults. (See Clark's Rule on page 197 to adjust dose appropriately for a child's weight.)

### LEMON BALM (*Melissa officinalis*)

Lemon balm supports heart and skin health, balances mood, calms an anxious mind, and repels insects. It is an effective carminative and when applied topically, it heals sores and lesions associated with herpes simplex. The essential oil of lemon balm produces a sense of calm in anxious children and reduces agitation in people with

Alzheimer's disease. Use a diffuser to disperse the essential oil of lemon balm in bedrooms or patios or gently simmer a handful of fresh or dried leaves in water to diffuse the aroma in the kitchen. To make a tea, take 2 teaspoons of fresh leaves and steep in 2 cups of water for 15 minutes, strain, and drink daily or as desired.

## LESSER CELANDINE (*Ficaria verna*)

Also known as pilewort, lesser celandine belongs to the buttercup family and is used topically for the treatment of skin ulcers and hemorrhoids. An ointment can be applied to the perineum after childbirth and suppositories can be made for hemorrhoids.

CAUTION: The plant should be dried prior to use to avoid contact dermatitis, and it should not be used internally.

### ⇥ *Lesser Celandine Suppositories for Hemorrhoids* ⇤

To make a rectal suppository, place ¼ cup of unrefined cocoa butter and ¼ cup of unrefined coconut oil in a double boiler and allow them to melt together, gently mixing. Add 2 tablespoons of powdered, previously dried lesser celandine and mix well. Strain, pour into a suppository mold, and freeze. (Some herbalists suggest using a homemade aluminum foil suppository mold, but it is best to avoid introducing aluminum into your mix.) The suppositories will keep in the freezer for 3 months, and they can also be applied to the skin as an ointment; however test this first as some people can experience contact dermatitis.

## LICORICE (*Glycyrrhiza glabra*)

Licorice is one of the most important herbs in Ayurvedic, Chinese Medicine, and American Indian medicine. The root of the licorice plant is rich in minerals, including sodium, potassium, iron, and manganese. It also contains glycyrrhizin, which increases cortisol production and inhibits its breakdown, making licorice effective in the treatment of adrenal fatigue. Because glycyrrhizin is also an antiviral, it suppresses the herpes virus internally and externally. A licorice gel can be applied to post-herpetic (shingles) neuralgia.

Licorice is especially useful in addressing infertility due to hormonal imbalance, polycystic ovary syndrome (PCOS), and menopausal symptoms, as well as fibromyalgia, chronic fatigue syndrome, and arteriosclerosis. Because licorice is soothing to the mucous membranes in the lungs, it is useful for people who smoke or are in the process of quitting. Licorice is an important herb for treating GERD and gastric ulcers. It is also used in Chinese Medicine to reduce the toxicity of certain herbs.

A typical recommended dose is drinking a decoction of the root 3 times a day. Make the decoction by placing 1 to 5 grams of the herb into 1½ cups of water and simmering, covered, for 10 to 15 minutes. Strain and drink.

CAUTION: Traditionally used in desert regions for its ability to help cells retain fluids, licorice is contraindicated for people with hypertension or edema. Higher doses ranging from 1 to 14 grams of glycyrrhizin can lead to increased hypertension and edema. I recommend that these individuals drink *no more than* 3 cups of tea a week, or they can use a deglycyrrhizinated product for GERD.

### LOBELIA (*Lobelia inflate*; *Campanulaceae*)

Known as Indian tobacco or pokeweed, lobelia is native to North America and is used as a tincture or tea to treat asthma, coughs, and bronchitis. It is also blended with kinnikinnick to inhale as smoke. Kinnikinnick is the name used by many American Indian communities and First Nations peoples to refer to a "smoking mix" and it is most often associated with the bearberry plant (*Arctostaphylos uva-ursi*). Lobelia is a powerful antispasmodic and an emetic, which in large quantities can be toxic. It is both a sedative and a stimulant, with psychoactive properties. It also contains lobeline, an alkaloid that acts as an antagonist to nicotinic receptors in the brain, making it useful for eliminating nicotine addiction. Thus, it is often combined with other nicotine withdrawal herbal compounds. (See "Protocol to Withdraw and Cease Nicotine Use" on page 139.) Lobelia is effective for nicotine withdrawal when used as a standardized tincture, 20 drops 4 times a day.

### MACA (*Lepidium meyenii*)

Maca, also called Peruvian ginseng, is rich in protein, natural sugars, calcium, fiber, iron, potassium, and iodine. The root is often called a super food that enhances libido and fertility. It also increases endurance and energy, helps relieve menopausal symptoms, regulates heavy and irregular periods, improves skin, and elevates mood. Fresh maca can be roasted, boiled, and mashed; however it is generally available as a powder and can be added to your smoothie. Take about 2,000 milligrams a day.

### MARJORAM (*Origanum majorana*) See page 125.

## MILK THISTLE (*Silybum marianum*)

Milk thistle is one of the most effective herbs for maintaining liver health and treating liver diseases. The active constituents are called silymarins, which have a strong antioxidant action and improve protein synthesis. Milk thistle is also used for blood-sugar regulation, diabetes, diabetic neuropathy, cirrhosis, hepatitis, and nonalcoholic fatty liver disease. It is an important herb in treating drug and alcohol recovery and for people who experience multiple chemical sensitivity syndromes. Veterinarians also prescribe milk thistle for dogs with liver disease or elevated liver enzymes. Milk thistle is often combined with the other liver herbs like dandelion and Oregon grape root. Do not use during pregnancy or lactation. Use the extract, capsules, or ground seeds in smoothies (recipe follows).

### ≫ *Happy Liver Smoothie* ≪

Chinese Medicine suggests that a sluggish liver makes a person angry, so if we enhance liver function, we reduce anger and improve our mood! This smoothie combines all the ingredients necessary to improve liver function. Lecithin (phosphatidylcholine) helps break down fat in the liver and improves brain function.

**MAKES 1 SERVING**

1 cup hemp or almond milk

1 teaspoon lecithin granules

1 to 2 teaspoons milk thistle
    seed powder

¾ cup frozen or fresh berries of
    your choice (blueberry, blackberry,
    raspberry)

Stevia or raw local honey (optional)

Add the ingredients to a blender and blend until combined. Drink once a day for 3 to 6 months. Test liver function for improvement using an ultrasound and a blood draw to test levels of liver enzymes.

## MINTS (*Lamiaceae*)

Spearmint and peppermint are the most commonly used therapeutic mints. Menthol, the primary volatile oil found in the mint family, gives the plant its unique aroma and its medicinal properties. Mints provide gentle support by helping to digest food, relieving flatulence and nausea, and soothing the digestive tract. Mint tea reduces nausea and vomiting during pregnancy. Mint oil can be applied externally to painful joints and muscles, after exercise, or for arthritis. A few drops of peppermint oil applied to the temples reduces tension headaches, and the aroma of peppermint elevates mood. Menthol is a powerful decongestant, and inhaling vapors from mints reduces congestion during colds and respiratory infections. Mint is also a nervine tonic. Drink a cup of mint tea after a meal to relax and enhance digestion.

### MORINGA (*Moringa oleifera*)

All of the parts of the moringa plant are used medicinally. It is rich in vitamins and minerals and is particularly high in iron and quercetin, which makes it valuable for treating allergies. The dried leaves are rich in protein and can be dried, powdered, and then sprinkled on cereals or salad.

Moringa has traditionally been used as a circulatory stimulant, antibacterial, antipyretic, anti-inflammatory, diuretic, antihypertensive, and antifungal. It is added to creams to enhance the appearance of skin. Moringa is often found in powdered or capsule form and can be added to your daily smoothie up to 4 grams a day.

### MOTHERWORT (*Leonurus cardiaca*)

Motherwort, meaning "mother's herb," is traditionally used as a uterine tonic, aiding every process related to the female reproductive system. It is used to ease childbirth, bring on a delayed labor, and reduce menstrual pains and menopausal symptoms. Motherwort also eases wheezing, coughing, and bronchitis, improves heart function, and reduces hormonally mediated stress and anxiety. It's pretty bitter so is best taken as a tincture, 4 to 12 milliliters daily (1:5 at 45%).

CAUTION: Motherwort is contraindicated for people who are pregnant or have endometriosis or fibroids.

### MUGWORT (*Artemisia vulgaris*)

A magical plant, mugwort is found in almost every traditional medicine system in the world. A tea made from the leaves functions as a diuretic, digestive tonic, mild sedative, and reproductive tonic. It is a powerful uterine stimulant, bringing on delayed menstruation and delayed afterbirth, and it eases symptoms of menopause. It is also a diaphoretic and febrifuge, making it useful during fevers and colds.

Mugwort is used in moxibustion, which is the process of burning mugwort on or just above certain acupuncture points on the body. Moxibustion is particularly helpful as an analgesic. Burning mugwort as an incense in the home is soothing and burning it outside repels mosquitoes. It is available in cone, stick, or as a loose plant.

You can also make a strong mugwort tea as a final rinse for the hair and skin following bathing.

CAUTION: Because mugwort is also an abortifacient, it is contraindicated in pregnancy.

### MULLEIN (*Verbascum thapsus*)

Mullein is a fuzzy-leafed plant typically prepared as an infusion to treat lung infections and congestion. It acts as an expectorant and demulcent, making it an essential medicine for coughs, bronchitis, chronic obstructive pulmonary disease, and asthma. Mullein (and garlic) eardrops are effective remedies for ear infections. The oil from the seeds and flowers, which contain saponins and mucopolysaccharides, are used for topical applications and the mucilage content in mullein makes it an appropriate external application for skin inflammation. Let a teaspoon of flowers and leaves steep in 1 cup of just-boiled water and drink 2 cups daily for a cough.

### MUSK MALLOW (*Malva moschata*)

A staple of Chinese cuisine, musk mallow flowers, seeds, and leaves are all edible. It is a very gentle plant with no adverse effects, and it is a beautiful plant to grow in the garden. Medicinally, the powdered seeds are used for dental pain, digestive complaints, heart health, and respiratory and urinary infections. The plant's demulcent properties reduce inflammation internally and externally. An infusion can be used as an eyewash, and poultices made from the leaves and flowers can be applied to bruises, cuts, and insect bites. It can also be a gentle laxative for young children. I like to make a strong infusion and keep it in the fridge where I can use it internally and topically as needed. Take 1 tablespoon of the dried flowers and leaves (2 tablespoons if using fresh). Pour 2 cups of hot water over and let it sit 15 minutes. Then strain, cool, and store for a week in the fridge. If you use it as an eyewash, make sure you strain it through very fine cheesecloth or an unbleached muslin bag twice.

### MUSTARD (*Brassica juncea*; *Brassica nigra*; *Sinapis alba*) *See* page 125.

### NETTLE (*Urtica*; *Urtica dioica*)

Also known as stinging nettle, this herbaceous perennial appears in early spring, growing in large patches in moist and shady areas. Both the leaves and stem are covered in hair-like needles that sting on contact.

Among the Chehalis people, nettle is called *qwunqwu'n*, meaning "it stings you." Nettle leaf is rich in chlorophyll, nutrients, and minerals. Phytochemicals found in stinging nettle are as follows: histamine, acetylcholine, serotonin, flavonol glycosides, beta-sitosterol, lectin, coumarins, hydroxysitosterol, scopoletin, tannins, and lignans. Nettle is stimulating for the bladder and kidneys, acting as a diuretic and anti-inflammatory. It also helps to remove excess uric acid making it useful for treating gout.

Nettle leaves and plant tips should be collected with gloves and scissors when they are about eight inches high and before they flower in the spring. The leaves can also be gathered in late spring and summer and used to make tea.

New nettles also come up in the fall and can be harvested before the first frost. Nettles make an excellent spring tonic, and oils and ointments are useful in treating skin problems and arthritic or rheumatic pain. People with arthritis sometimes choose to pick stinging nettles without gloves because the "sting" they experience reduces pain. Nettles act as a counter-irritant and rubifacient due to the formic acid and histamine contained within that causes the stinging sensation and then leads to pain relief. If you want the same results but without the stinging pain, use an extract of anti-inflammatory hox alpha, which is extracted from nettles and is currently available in Germany.

Drink a stinging nettle infusion or tea daily. To make it fresh, simply soak the whole leaves—fresh or dried—in just-boiled water for 10 to 20 minutes, strain, and enjoy. No sweetener required. You can also steam the leaves and add some oil to them or take a tincture of the plant.

## OATS AND OAT STRAW (*Avena sativa*)

The fresh buds of oats contain milky seedpods, which are responsible for the grass's most potent medicinal qualities. Oats and milk oat seeds are powerful nervines, and the young shoots nourish and restore a body and mind under stress. Topically, oat grain or oat straw is a soothing wash for external use for itchy irritation and inflammation of the skin and can be added to soaking baths. Oats contain calcium, iron, magnesium, and high-soluble fiber content and make a relaxing meal in the evening in contrast to breakfast when they are usually eaten. Young milky oats are best used as a tincture, 3 to 15 milliliters daily, whereas oat straw is best taken as a fresh infusion totaling 5 to 15 grams daily.

⇥ *Fresh Oat Milk* ⇤

Oat milk is a healthy alternative to cow's milk since many people are sensitive or allergic to bovine dairy. It's naturally relaxing and can be used in smoothies or on cereal.

**MAKES 4 CUPS**

Soak 1 cup of rolled oats in water overnight. Strain the oats (option: save the soaking water for a soothing poultice or bath for itchy skin) and add them to 4 cups of water and blend. Then strain again through a nut milk bag or cheesecloth, bottle, and refrigerate for up to 4 days.

---

### OREGON GRAPE ROOT (*Berberis aquifolium*)

Oregon grape root is a must-have medicine for skin and digestive health. Closely related to the barberry plant and rich in berberine, it lowers blood glucose in people with diabetes. It is also a liver stimulant that activates the production of bile, and it loosens and expels waste in the digestive tract. Oregon grape root is used topically to treat psoriasis and atopic dermatitis and is often used as a substitute for the endangered wild goldenseal. Make an infusion using 1 teaspoon of dried root gently simmered in 1 cup of water for 20 minutes, strain, and drink 1 cup a day. Use the tea or extract short-term only (2 to 4 weeks) as needed.

### OSHA ROOT, BEAR ROOT (*Ligusticum*; *Ligusticum porter*)

Osha root is an aromatic bitter in the carrot family that is used for upper respiratory infections and as an expectorant. Upon waking from hibernation, bears seek out the root and rub it on their bodies to stimulate their appetite, thus the name "bear root." Popular among indigenous peoples in the United States, osha root stimulates menses, increases circulation, and promotes sweating. The root is eaten as a mild digestive, as the bitterness helps indigestion and flatulence. Because osha is difficult to domesticate, nearly all osha root on the market is harvested in the wild. Among the Zuni people, both the medicine person and the patient chew the root during healing ceremonies. Use a tincture of the fresh root (1:2), 20 to 40 drops up to 5 times daily or make a decoction by adding a large handful of root to 3 cups of boiling water on the stove top and simmering for 6 hours. You will have about 2 cups of decocted osha and can drink 1 to 2 cups a day or add ½ cup to a smoothie over several days.

### PARTRIDGE (*Mitchella repens*)

The berries of the partridge vine are a woman's ally. They can be used as an emmenagogue, parturient, and styptic. A tea is used for painful menstrual cramps, infertility, UTIs, and interstitial cystitis. Note that the tea can be taken in the few weeks before childbirth but not during the early weeks of pregnancy. Partridge berries' astringent and diuretic qualities make them useful for diarrhea, and a wash or salve made from the whole plant can be used topically for sore or cracked breasts from breastfeeding.

**PASSIONFLOWER** (*Passiflora*; *Passiflora edulis*) *See* page 137.

**PLANTAIN** (*Plantago*; *Plantago major*)

The *Plantago* genus has 250 species, but the one most commonly referred to is common plantain or *Plantago major*. The plant is effective externally as a vulnerary, and internally as an astringent and anti-inflammatory. The plant's active compounds include iridoids such as aucubin and catalpol, the flavonoids apigenin and luteolin, tannins, and oleanolic acids. A tea of the leaves suppresses coughs and is a gentle expectorant that soothes mucous membranes. Plantain also helps diarrhea, IBS, hemorrhoids, and ulcers, as it is both astringent and cooling. The seeds of the plant are laxative, containing 30 percent mucilage that expands in the gut, easing the passage of waste. Externally, the plant is a styptic and soothes irritated and inflamed skin. It is also applied to the temples as an analgesic for headaches. It can be taken as a tea or tincture, and an ointment, poultice, or salve can be applied externally.

**RED CLOVER** (*Trifolium pratense*)

Red clover is rich in isoflavones and reduces the vasomotor symptoms of menopause such as hot flashes, as well as vaginal atrophy and dryness. It is also used for osteoporosis. Its main uses, traditionally, have been in the topical treatment of skin disorders, including psoriasis and eczema. Doses range from 40 to 80 milligrams a day of red clover isoflavone extract, with the higher dose found to beneficially affect menopausal symptoms.

**RED RASPBERRY** (*Rubus idaeus*)

The raspberry plant has been used for millennia as a tonic for fertility, labor, and pregnancy. It strengthens the uterus, maintains healthy egg production in the ovaries, eases the pain of labor, and reduces the nausea and vomiting associated with pregnancy. Red raspberry leaf is rich in quercetin, a natural antihistamine and decongestant for allergies. Quercetin also supports lung and heart health, promotes a stable blood pressure, and keeps inflammation down. Red raspberry leaf can be used as an infusion or extract.

**REHMANNIA ROOT** (*Rehmannia glutinosa*)

Rehmannia root, also referred to as Chinese foxglove, is an effective kidney and adrenal tonic. This Chinese Medicine adaptogen is restorative and nourishing to overworked adrenals and kidneys and is an excellent tonic for chronic fatigue. It is also used for Alzheimer's and Parkinson's diseases and for lowering blood sugar in type 2 diabetes. The dried root prepared as a decoction is the preferred mode of ingestion. Doses range from 5 to 30 grams a day.

### RHODIOLA (*Sedum roseum*)

Rhodiola is an important adaptogen used to lift mood, reduce anxiety and depression, and improve physical and mental performance. It increases stamina by increasing the red blood cell count and lowering oxidative damage and shortens the recovery time after long workouts. It also boosts mental clarity, concentration, and sexual function and encourages restful sleep. It is used as a substitute for coffee. Rhodiola increases serotonin, dopamine, and opioid peptide levels and benefits cognitive functioning. Rosavin, rhodiola's primary active compound, helps normalize cortisol levels and burn fat.

Rhodiola is a very gentle yet potent botanical, making it especially useful for someone who can use only one botanical or who has multiple chemical sensitivities. It is also an ideal botanical for the treatment of traumatic stress.

For fatigue associated with stress, start with of 10 drops of extract 4 times a day and gradually increase to 30 drops, 3 to 4 times a day. For memory, concentration, and enhanced cognition take 100 to 400 milligrams a day using a standardized extract containing at least 3 percent rosavin extract or make a tea from the roots. No serious side effects have been reported, but rhodiola can be stimulating, so it should be used earlier in the day. People who develop mania in response to antidepressants could respond similarly to high doses of rhodiola. Individuals who are anxious may feel jittery or agitated. If this occurs, then a smaller dose with very gradual increases may be needed.

### ROSELLE, JAMAICA (*Hibiscus sabdariffa*)

Roselle is a medicinal hibiscus flower. It is commonly called Jamaica (pronounced ha-myka in Spanish) throughout Mexico, and it is believed to have been introduced to the Western Hemisphere in the 1700s by African slaves and brought to Jamaica—hence the name. Jamaica makes a delicious bright red drink that is a very accessible and inexpensive source of vitamin C, calcium, and powerful antioxidants. Its polyphenol compounds are similar to those found in blueberry, cranberry, cherry, and blackberry.

It is most often found in Mexican and Central American markets in the United States. The calyces of the Jamaica plant are used traditionally as a refreshing beverage called *agua de Jamaica*. It is also used traditionally in Mexico as a medicine to reduce fever during colds and to provide nourishment during illness. It also lowers cholesterol and blood glucose, reduces risk of heart disease, has hypotensive (lowers blood pressure) and antibacterial activity, and is protective of kidneys and the liver. In addition, Jamaica has high levels of anthocyanins, powerful antioxidants that scavenge inflammatory cells in the body. To gain medicinal benefits, drink 1 to 2 glasses of Jamaica daily (recipe follows).

---

⇉ *Roselle Tea/Agua de Jamaica* ⇇

**MAKES 4 CUPS**

Boil 1 quart of water and add a heaping handful of Jamaica calyces. Gently simmer for 10 minutes until richly red. Strain and add a little honey or stevia to taste. Note: do not add sugar, as it counteracts the effects of the natural antioxidants. Jamaica makes a wonderful drink, hot or cold. Add a tablespoon of collagen powder when it is cold to make it a meal.

---

**ROSEMARY (*Rosmarinus officinalis*) See page 127.**

**RUE (*Ruta graveolens*)**
Rue is an ornamental plant that has a strong smell and bitter taste. It is native to Europe, and it is also found in kitchen gardens throughout tropical regions and temperate zones in the Southern Hemisphere. Rue is used to relieve pain, especially headaches, and promote menstruation. In culinary dishes the leaves are used fresh or dried for seasoning fish and salads. It flavors liquors and because of its bitterness, provides the tonic properties of a perfect digestive to drink after eating a heavy meal. Rue is used worldwide in traditional medicine to induce abortion and also as an emmenagogue. Typically, rue is taken in the form of an extract or tea. Take a few small sprigs and pour a cup of boiling water over them and let it sit for 5 minutes. Drink 1 cup a day as needed. Rue is also an effective insect repellent.

**SAGE (*Salvia*; *Salvia apiana*; *Salvia officinalis*)**
White sage (*Salvia apiana*) is a sacred plant, native in North America. Sacred sage has a sweet smell and is often bundled and burned ceremonially to cleanse and purify people and places. Traditionally a tea is made to provide strength after giving

birth. Its overuse and overharvesting by non-native peoples have led to concerns about cultural appropriation of traditional native ceremonies leading to resource depletion.

Common sage (*Salvia officinalis*), from Europe, is used to flavor foods, as a tea to improve mood, and as a calming essential oil. Sage tea calms gastrointestinal distress, reduces night sweats during menopause, and is an effective emmenagogue. A strong sage tea can be used as a mouth rinse to heal gingivitis.

### SARSAPARILLA (*Smilax*)

Various species of the *Smilax* genus have been used in a number of ways. *Smilax ornata*, also called Jamaican sarsaparilla, which is commonly found in Mexico and Central America, is the base of a root beer called sarsaparilla. When it was introduced to the New World, this species was the primary treatment for syphilis. The *Smilax aristolochiifolia* species, native to Mexico and Central America, is used as an aphrodisiac and for its progestogenic qualities. A root tea is made to improve digestion and appetite and build lean body mass, and the stems of the plant can be used to treat toothaches. It is also used in extract or capsule form as an anti-inflammatory.

### SAVORY (*Satureja hortensis*) See page 128.

### SCHISANDRA (*Schisandra chinensis*)

Schisandra is also called the Five Flavor Berry because the fruit tastes sweet, sour, salty, bitter, and hot, all at the same time. Part of the magnolia vine family, the fruits and leaves of this woody vine can be consumed as food or taken medicinally. The berry is one of the most important medicines in Asian Traditional Medicines and is used as an adaptogen or as a tonic to prevent or treat fatigue. Schisandra should be used as part of any adrenal fatigue recovery program and for optimal mental function. It is listed in the Russian official pharmacopoeia, as it has been widely researched and used for whole-system health. Similar to ginseng, schisandra is used for longevity and physical endurance. The lignans in the plant help to regenerate liver tissue that has been damaged from alcohol abuse and are also neuroprotective and therefore should be a foundational herb in the prevention and treatment of cognitive decline.

I love the bright red of these berries and often mix them with a few roselle petals to supercharge my energy and mental focus or to give me an immune boost if I have a cough or cold. Use it as a tea, capsule, tincture, or liquid extract, make a schisandra syrup or cordial (recipe follows), or eat the berries fresh. Take 500 milligrams in capsules, twice daily.

CAUTION: Not for use by people with ulcers or epilepsy.

---

→ *Schisandra Cordial* ←

**MAKES 3 CUPS**

1 cup dried schisandra berries

1 quart water

½ cup raw local honey

½ cup brandy

In a large pot over low heat, gently simmer the berries in the water until the liquid is reduced to about a pint. This may take several hours. Strain, put the mixture back into the pot over very low heat, and add in the honey, stirring until it is blended. Make sure you don't boil the mixture, as it removes the benefits of the honey. Cool, add the brandy, and bottle. Keep in the fridge for up to 3 months and take a tablespoon midafternoon for a pick-me-up.

---

## SEA PLANTS/SEA VEGETABLES/SEAWEEDS

Sea plants, often called seaweeds, are large algae that grow in almost any body of water. They are classified as green, brown, or red, have more nutrients and vitamins than any land vegetable, and are rich in antioxidants and high in soluble fiber. They are the most effective plants in supporting thyroid function because of their high iodine content. Kombu (*Saccharina*), wakame (*Undaria pinnatifida*), dulse (*Palmaria palmata*), kelp (order *Laminariales*), and nori (*Pyropia*) are the most popular species of seaweed generally seen in grocery stores.

The easiest way to consume seaweed is to include it in your daily diet. Seaweed herbal salt combinations are available to season food, and packaged seaweed can also be purchased. Note that they usually come dehydrated, and you must soak the leaves before cooking. Seaweed tablets or capsules with sodium alginate are also available and used to eliminate heavy metals from the body. Finally, seaweeds make wonderful facials and skin treatments and can be added to a bath for relaxation and pain relief.

### → Seaweed Detoxification ←

Algins in brown algae remove heavy metals from the body. Most heavy metal toxicity is absorbed via exposed foods, air pollution, or industrial chemicals, fertilizers, and pesticides as well as from swimming pools and spas treated with chlorine and halides. Conducting a tissue mineral analysis on the hair can show what heavy metals are being excreted through the hair.

After I soak seaweed for my recipes, I save the liquid and add it to my soup or give my dog a teaspoonful in his food. If you want an additional option for detoxifying with seaweed, I was introduced to this protocol by Dr. Nicholas Gonzalez, the esteemed immunologist as part of his detoxification protocols for cancer patients.

Take a capsule of sodium alginate 3 times a day between meals for 5 days, every 3 months.

### SELF-HEAL (*Prunella vulgaris*)

Self-heal, or heal-all, is also called Heart of the Earth and is another "cure-all" herb that is regarded in Chinese Medicine as a plant that can change the course of a disease. It also provides edible leaves and stems when young. It is an effective lymphatic cleanser, antiviral (particularly against the herpes simplex virus), and wound healer. It staunches the bleeding of wounds, burns, and ulcers, supports the gastrointestinal tract, and helps decrease inflammation in Crohn's disease. Self-heal contains immunomodulating polysaccharides, which support a healthy immune system. These actions, paired with lymphatic cleansing, make it an excellent treatment for allergies. Self-heal is also used to treat fevers, thyroid dysfunction, hepatitis, jaundice, high blood pressure, and edema. Steep 1 teaspoon of dried herb in 1 cup of water for 20 minutes and drink 2 cups a day for 1 week for acute illness. This protocol can also be used daily for several months to address chronic inflammatory conditions.

### SENNA, CANDLE BUSH (*Senna alexandrina*; *Senna alata*)

Popular in Ayurvedic medicine, senna is a potent laxative used for constipation. It causes contractions in the intestinal tract, resulting in elimination of waste from the bowels. The contractions are a result of anthraquinones in the plant leaves. A liquid extract or a tablet of senna is the most popular way to consume the plant, though it is available as a tea. Senokot and Ex-Lax are commercial laxatives containing senna and are available in pharmacies. Senna should be used only on occasion, as the cause of constipation should be treated.

### SHATAVARI (*Asparagus racemosus*)

*Shatavari* means "woman who has a hundred husbands," which likely refers to the plant's ability to strengthen the female reproductive system. Shatavari is a type of asparagus found throughout Nepal, Sri Lanka, and India. It is an excellent herb for female infertility used in both Ayurvedic medicine and also found in the British pharmacopoeia. It is taken to prevent miscarriage and menopausal symptoms, for PCOS and to increase breast milk and libido. It also treats ulcers, hyperacidity in the stomach, and bronchial infections and supports overall immune system function. The root is typically processed and then dried and can be taken as a decoction or powder or added to ghee. Externally, the root can be applied to treat stiff joints. Herb menstruum ratio is 1:5: add 20 drops to 1 to 2 ounces of water up to 4 times a day or take a 500 milligram capsule twice a day.

### SHEPHERD'S PURSE (*Capsella bursa-pastoris*)

Shepherd's purse is a potent uterine tonic used for heavy menstrual bleeding. Topically, the herb has been used to staunch bleeding and heal wounds. The plant is also used as an anti-inflammatory and antibacterial, and it supports fertility and decreases the pain and stiffness associated with rheumatoid arthritis. Drink a shepherd's purse infusion or take a tincture every day for 4 days before the start of menstruation to reduce a heavy menstrual flow.

### SKULLCAP, AMERICAN (*Scutellaria lateriflora*)

American skullcap is a nervine and antispasmodic. It is used to treat exhaustion, anxiety, restlessness, and tension, and it gently aids stress and insomnia. American skullcap is hepatoprotective, antioxidant, anticonvulsant, antibacterial, and antiviral. It relaxes and soothes uterine tissue and is beneficial in supporting lung function in pneumonia. Make a tea of skullcap before bed by adding a teaspoon of fresh or dried flowers to a cup of water, or take a 500 to 800 milligram capsule.

### SKULLCAP, CHINESE (*Scutellaria baicalensis*)

Not to be confused with American skullcap, the dried roots of Chinese skullcap are called *huang qin* (meaning "golden herb") and are one of the most important herbal medicines in Asia. A decoction or tincture is used for hypertension, diarrhea, respiratory infections, insomnia, pain, chronic inflammation, and protection of brain neurons. Baicalein, baicalin, and wogonoside are the flavones that give the plant some of its strong therapeutic qualities. The herb is hepatoprotective and used to treat hepatitis. It is also an antibacterial, antiviral, and antioxidant. Combined with catechu (Acacia catechu), it decreases pain and inflammation. Take a 500 milligram capsule, 1 to 2 times a day.

## SLIPPERY ELM (*Ulmus rubra*)

A must to have on hand for its extensive application, the inner bark of the slippery elm contains a mucilaginous fiber that soothes any inflammation externally or internally. It is a common ingredient in various throat lozenges. The tea is indicated for throat irritation and is an excellent remedy for digestive complaints, including gastritis, colitis, ulcers, inflammation of the intestinal tract, upset stomach, and diarrhea. It also soothes inflammation in the respiratory and urinary tracts. Slippery elm is also very nutritious and can be eaten as porridge; however, due to its growing endangered status, it is not commonly used this way. The bark of slippery elm is available in powdered form and can be made into a paste and applied topically for skin irritations or used in a tea (recipe follows).

### » *Slippery Elm Bark Tea* «

**MAKES 2½ CUPS**

Gently simmer 2 heaping tablespoons of bark or powder in 3 cups of water for 20 minutes. Let sit, reheat, and then strain. Drink the tea up to 3 times a day and save the material that does not pass through the strainer to use topically as a poultice.

## SOAPBERRIES (*Sapindus*)

Soapberries, or soap nuts, are the fruits of a small genus of shrubs. They are used by native peoples in the United States and Canada to make "Indian ice cream," which is a frothy foam dessert mixed with berries. Soapberries are also used to treat high blood pressure, clear acne, and induce labor. A decoction of the inner bark of the shrub is an effective laxative and can be used as a digestive tonic. Applied topically, a wash or rinse can be used as an eyewash for pinkeye or sties and to help heal cuts, swellings, sores, and ulcers. Soapberries can also be ground into a powder and added to cleaning solutions like shampoo, laundry detergent, and face or dish soap.

### SOY (*Glycine max*)

Soy is among one of the most controversial plants when it comes to discussions of its positive or negative effects on women's health. Soy is high in isoflavones, a type of phytoestrogen that, when interacting with estrogen receptors in the human body, can result in either estrogenic or antiestrogenic activity. Factors that affect soy's activity in the body include existing hormone levels and imbalances, whether one is premenopausal or postmenopausal, and the types of soy products consumed and whether they are fermented or highly processed. Soy is also a trypsin inhibitor, which depresses thyroid function and is thought by some researchers to have a carcinogenic effect.

When I am making decisions on controversial research for myself and my patients, I ask how the plant is used in traditional, authentic diets in order to gain insight into indigenous knowledge systems. If we study the soy used in Asia, we find that it is most often fermented. Fermentation "predigests" soy, breaking down the enzyme inhibitors that lead to side effects. We do not see soy burgers or soy protein isolate additives used in traditional Asian food. The verdict? Small amounts of fermented soy products like shoyu, miso, and natto will generally be fine for most women; however women with cancer or at higher risk for hormone-based cancers, digestive problems, pancreatitis, and hypothyroidism should avoid soy.

### STAR ANISE (*Illicium verum*) *See* page 128.

### STILLINGIA (*Stillingia sylvatica*)

Called Queen's Delight, the fresh root of the stillingia plant, while rarely used today, is one of the most effective cleansing and detoxifying herbs. The root is a powerful alterative that supports natural detoxification of the mucous membranes, liver, and lymphatic tissue and removes toxins from the body. It is also an effective expectorant and used for fevers and constipation. Large quantities can cause vomiting. The fresh root simmered in a cup of tea or tincture of the root is the most effective way to ingest the plant. Stillingia tea can be made from ½ teaspoon of dried root added to a cup of boiled water. Drink 1 to 2 cups a day for up to 2 weeks. Combine with external skin brushing when a lymphatic cleanse is required.

### TAMARIND (*Tamarindus indica*) *See* page 129.

### TEA, BLACK (*Camellia sinensis*)

Black tea and green tea are the same plant. However, black tea is fermented and is rich in theaflavin antioxidants. Like green tea, black tea can give a mood and energy boost and helps weight loss by breaking down fats. Teas vary in flavor depending on where they are grown, the type of soil they are grown in, and fermenting conditions. Teas bags may be moistened and applied to puffy eyes to reduce swelling. Earl Grey is a black tea flavored with essential oil of bergamot, which is known to be a healing herb for the heart.

### TEA, GREEN (*Camellia sinensis*)

Green tea has been studied extensively for its remarkable abilities to reduce the risks of age-related cognitive impairment. Green tea contains both caffeine and L-theanine. Caffeine improves cognition, mood, and memory, while L-theanine synergistically works with the caffeine to create a milder stimulant with longer sustained energy. L-theanine also increases both the gamma-aminobutyric acid (GABA) function in the brain, causing an anxiolytic effect, and the production of alpha waves in the brain, which leads to a meditative state without slowing the brain down. Antioxidants in green tea reduce the risk of cancers and cardiovascular disease. Green tea's catechin compounds have various benefits—from protecting the brain from Alzheimer's and Parkinson's to lowering the risk of certain infections from viruses and diseases and improving dental health. Green tea powder can be added to your daily smoothie and there are many varieties of loose-leaf teas to explore. I especially like drinking different types of loose-leaf sencha. Drink 2 to 3 cups a day.

### THYME (*Thymus vulgaris*) *See* page 129.

### TRIBULUS (*Tribulus terrestris*)

Used in Ayurvedic medicine, tribulus, also called bindii, increases libido in women. A regular intake of tribulus also reduces hot flashes and depression during menopause. It can also be used for symptoms related to PMS. A concentrated dose of 60 percent saponin extract should range between 100 and 300 milligrams a day.

### TRIPHALA (*Terminalia chebula*; *Phyllanthus emblica*; *Terminalia bellirica*)

Triphala is a traditional Ayurvedic formula that contains three fruits native to India that work synergistically to support healthy respiratory, urinary, cardiovascular, reproductive, and urinary systems. Because it facilitates proper digestion and elimination, triphala is also used as a mild laxative and part of a weight-loss protocol. The taste of triphala is an important part of its healing and sipping and savoring a tea is especially useful for weight loss. The best time to take triphala is on an empty stomach, upon waking and right before bed. It can be used as a tea, liquid extract, or as a capsule of 1,500 to 2,000 milligrams daily in 2 divided doses.

### TURMERIC (*Curcuma longa*)

Turmeric is a powerful antioxidant and anti-inflammatory used for rheumatoid arthritis, menstrual cramps, digestive complaints, musculoskeletal pain, and dementia prevention. It is also used for gallbladder health and pancreatitis. Combine 100 to 200 milligrams of turmeric with 5 grams of glutamine daily for treatment of ulcerative colitis. The bioavailability of curcumin, the primary active substance in turmeric, is potentiated by fat and piperine, a compound found in black pepper and fat, so the use of turmeric should combine both. The fresh root can be juiced and added to smoothies or used in daily cooking.

## » *Golden Milk* «

This healing beverage is a variation on the traditional Ayurvedic recipe. I drink it hot in the winter and over ice during the summer.

**MAKES 1 SERVING**

1 teaspoon coconut oil

¾ teaspoon ground turmeric

⅛ teaspoon freshly ground black pepper

¼ teaspoon ground ashwagandha

2 drops vanilla extract, or ⅛ teaspoon ground vanilla

⅛ teaspoon ground cardamom

⅛ teaspoon ground cinnamon bark

¼ teaspoon ground dried dates

Pinch of sea salt (optional)

1 cup coconut, cashew, or almond milk

Mix all the dry ingredients together and then warm the milk in a small saucepan over low heat. Add the mix to the warm milk and froth it to ensure a blend. When it is hot, pour and enjoy.

### USNEA (*Usnea*)

*Usnea* is a genus of lichen: a combination of algae and fungus that grows on trees. It can be used externally and internally as an antifungal, antibacterial, and antimicrobial. It is used in Chinese Medicine, American Indian medicine, and throughout Mexico and South America. While usnea has been used both internally and externally without side effects, its active constituent, usnic acid, when extracted and concentrated and used for weight loss at high doses, has been implicated in hepatic failure, suggesting that usnea should be used under the guidance of a skilled herbalist. The lichen is also used as a dye and for sanitary wound dressings and for making diapers. Usnea can be made into a salve, a tincture, or a lozenge. The German Commission E suggests lozenges with preparations equivalent to 100 millgrams of the herb can be used 3 to 6 times a day. Its use should be limited to between 7 and 10 days.

### UVA URSI (*Arctostaphylos uva-ursi*)

Uva ursi, or bearberry, treats urinary tract inflammation due to bacteria. The leaves of the bearberry plant have been shown to destroy several strains of bacteria and fungi. The arbutin in the plant turns into hydroquinone in the urinary tract, which then acts as a natural antibiotic. Uva ursi is indicated for women who have recurring episodes of UTIs or chronic cystitis. Known also as kinnikinnick, it is a component of a smoking mixture used ceremonially by native peoples in the United States and Canada.

### VALERIAN (*Valeriana officinalis*) *See* page 140.

### VERVAIN (*Verbena officinalis*)

The leaves and the roots of vervain have diverse applications including use as an antidiarrheal, analgesic, anthelmintic, astringent, diaphoretic, emmenagogue, expectorant, vermifuge, and vulnerary. It is a relaxing nervine with an affinity for the liver and gallbladder. Vervain is helpful for irritability, mood swings, depression, and anxiety and can enhance dreams and act as an aphrodisiac. It can act as an abortifacient so should be avoided during pregnancy. It is also used as a mouth gargle or wash for sore throats and bleeding gums. A tea can be made from fresh or dried leaves by placing ¼ cup (dried) or ½ cup (fresh) in boiled water.

### WATERCRESS (*Nasturtium officinale*)

Watercress is a super plant because of its high nutritional and mineral content with powerful antioxidant and anti-inflammatory properties. It has a peppery bite that mixes well with fat to benefit the liver. It prevents bruising, improves the appearance of skin, and helps reduce inflammation in eczema. Watercress can be juiced, added to salads, or made into a soup to reduce respiratory mucus.

### WHITE WILLOW (*Salix alba*)

The bark of the white willow tree contains the glycoside salicin, the compound that led to the discovery of aspirin. When ingested, salicin converts into salicylic acid, which is a cooling anti-inflammatory and analgesic. While slower acting than aspirin, it tends to work for a longer period and with fewer side effects. A tea or extract can be made from the inner bark, and a dose of standardized extract can provide up to 120 to 240 milligrams salicin per day in 4 to 6 doses.

### WILD YAM (*Dioscorea villosa*)

Wild yam is a relaxing herb used for the treatment of muscle and abdominal pain and poor circulation. It is also used as a uterine antispasmodic and tonic, which helps with painful menses and menopausal symptoms, and it can stimulate liver and pancreatic function. While wild yam is a healing plant for women, it does not have progesterone or estrogen activity. Although the constituents extracted from wild yam were once used to create pharmaceutical progesterone in a laboratory setting, the human body is unable to convert these plant constituents into precursors for sex hormones, so wild yam creams are not a good progesterone source. Instead, consider oral micronized progesterone or prescribed bioidentical progesterone cream.

### WITCH HAZEL (*Hamamelis*; *Hamamelis virginiana*)

The leaves and bark of the witch hazel tree are commonly prepared into astringent, cooling agents. Indigenous Americans use witch hazel for inflammatory skin conditions and skin injuries. It can be used for sores, bruises, psoriasis, bug bites, skin burns, varicose veins, hemorrhoids, and eczema. It is indicated for women post-childbirth to soothe and reduce swelling around the vaginal area. Make your own extract or purchase an organic witch hazel extract that has less that 20 percent alcohol.

### WOOD BETONY (*Stachys officinalis*)

A mild, gentle herb, wood betony is a nervine and muscle relaxant. It helps to relieve tension and stress and can be used at the onset of migraines. This herb stimulates and relaxes—boosting the body's vital energy while increasing resilience. It is helpful for calming obsessive thinking, anxiety, and PTSD. Wood betony can also help to decrease abnormal uterine bleeding in women with PCOS.

### YARROW (*Achillea millefolium*)

An ancient herb, yarrow has a long history of healing internal and external wounds, and an infusion can be applied to wounds to staunch bleeding and activate healing. Yarrow tea is anti-inflammatory and analgesic and soothes digestion. It also gently reduces a fever, helps with loss of appetite, and reduces mild spasms of the gastrointestinal tract. A strong infusion can be added to a sitz bath to decrease pelvic cramping.

### YELLOW DOCK (*Rumex crispus*)

Dock is a gentle laxative, and when combined with dandelion, burdock, nettles, and cleaver, makes an effective detoxifying formula. Dock can serve as a digestive bitter and a strong decoction of the root can be applied topically to treat skin wounds and hemorrhoids. Yellow dock is particularly high in iron and can therefore help with heavy menstruation, pregnancy, and anemia. Because supplemental iron can be problematic, yellow dock is a good option. Yellow dock can be taken as decoction, using 2 to 4 grams of dried root up to 3 times a day, or as an extract, using 1 to 2 milliliters (1:5 at 45%) up to 3 times a day.

## CONCLUSION

Nature has provided us with an abundance of herbs, offering flowers, leaves, seeds, roots, and barks with which to craft our medicines. We may choose to make medicines traditionally, estimating measures and experimenting with combinations, or we may follow instructions based on established scientific formulas. There are numerous high-quality prepared herbal remedies available in capsules, extract, and dried form for purchase, or we may head to the forest or our own backyard to forage. I have explored in this chapter a diversity of options for you to choose from to suit your needs. Whatever herbs you choose to use, your knowledge will turn to practical wisdom as you listen to the myriad ways your body and mind respond to these gifts from the earth.

# → 5 ←

# SPICE MEDICINE

S pices are medicine! They are sensory nourishment. They contain volatile oils that transform our consciousness and bring us joy and contentment as they elevate our mood and help us to relax. An easy and effective way to integrate herbal medicine into your daily routine is to use spices in your cooking. Spices can be incorporated into your meals as an illness preventative, and they are a powerful support when using food as medicine for whole-health healing when you are ill.

I love to make my own spice mixtures from whole seeds, leaves, and roots on the spot for meals or in advance to use as medicine when I am feeling ill. I also bottle spices and mixtures, along with favorite recipes, as gifts for my friends and family on special occasions.

Preparing spice mixtures as a group activity with friends and family provides "kitchen lessons" (I also call these lessons "culinary pedagogy"—for the highfalutin or for those who want to incorporate this knowledge into schools and universities) as we share the history, geography, health, medicine, indigenous knowledge, and women's stories surrounding a particular spice or plant. After all, the history of global exploration (and colonization and resource extraction) can be told by following the routes of the spice trade and the exchanges of foods across borders and seas. Did you know that there would be no Szechuan spicy eggplant without the peppers from Mexico, or that the Italians did not have a red sauce before 1492 when tomatoes were brought from Mexico? All the world's different peoples with their many different cultures use spices. In this chapter we will explore some familiar and hopefully some novel spices and mixtures that will enhance your healing and culinary adventures.

# SPICES

Many of these spices will have one or more recipes, and some include a brief "lesson" to share with your family and friends.

### ALLSPICE (*Pimenta dioica*)

The dried, unripe berries of this tropical tree are referred to as allspice, pimenta, Jamaican pepper, or myrtle pepper. It was given the name "allspice" by the English in the seventeenth century because it had notes of cinnamon, nutmeg, juniper berries, peppers, and cloves. Allspice is the foundation of Caribbean cuisine. It is used to flavor Jamaican jerk seasoning, moles, curry powders, pickling mixes, sauces, sausages, cold cuts, and relishes. Allspice contains eugenol, a potent antibacterial and antiseptic, which may be why it is also used to cure and preserve meats. In Costa Rica, allspice is used to treat indigestion and diabetes. In Guatemala, the berries are crushed to treat bruises, sore joints, and muscles. In Ayurveda, allspice is used in the treatment of toothaches and respiratory congestion. Allspice is also a central ingredient in most Mexican mole sauces and Jamaican jerk seasoning. Note that the volatile oils of allspice evaporate very easily so buy small quantities and store the berries in an amber glass jar with a tight lid. The lessons and recipes provided here will help you explore this healing culinary spice.

## ⇛ *Spice Lesson* ⇐

During the American colonial era, Caribbean pirates popularized a dish called boucan or buccan, which was meat marinated with allspice berries. Among the Taíno people in the Caribbean, the pirates were referred to as the *boucaniers*, or buccaneers. Buccan is also related to what the Spanish called *barbacoa*, which later became "barbecue."

## ⇛ *Allspice Tea* ⇐

**MAKES 1 SERVING**

In Jamaica, a tea made from allspice berries is taken for colds, menstrual cramps, and upset stomach. Slightly crush 1 tablespoon of berries, simmer them for 15 minutes in 1 cup of boiling water, and strain. Drink 2 cups a day for up to 1 week as needed.

## ↠ *Chocolate Mole Sauce* ↞

In this recipe you will be working with allspice, chilies, and much more to achieve a divine combination of hot spicy chocolate that will awaken anything it touches, especially chicken, turkey, or even tofu.

The key to working with chilies is to understand that water only spreads the heat, whether it's in your mouth or on your hands, so if you eat something too spicy, grab a piece of bread or a spoonful of rice. My *comadre* Alicia taught me this simple trick to avoid the stinging effects of chilies' volatile oils: After working with chilies rub your hands through your hair (be sure not to rub your eyes!) so that the volatile oils are absorbed by your hair. Then you are ready to wash your hands with soap and water.

*Mole* means "sauce" in Mexico. Its consistency and uses reflect the joining of European and Mexican spices and food techniques. I was introduced to mole negro on my first trip to Oaxaca and it's been a mainstay in my kitchen ever since. While moles are not found in the western part of Mexico where I live, in recent years many Oaxaqueños travel north with their spectacular moles to share at outdoor festivals. Moles last, so make a batch to eat and freeze the rest. The warmth of the allspice and heat of the pepper will warm and nourish you on a cold day, or help you sweat it out on a hot one. Mole often has some bread or tortilla added but I left it out for our gluten-free friends. You will be so glad you pulled out the allspice for this special treat and for other ingredients like chilies, plantain, Mexican oregano (*Lippia graveolens*), and *canela* (Mexican cinnamon). For these ingredients go to your local Mexican food store or shop online.

My recipe is a combination of several I have come across throughout the years, beginning with the one from esteemed chef Diana Kennedy. Mole is very forgiving, so you can certainly experiment a bit.

**MAKES 8 CUPS (ENOUGH FOR 4 POUNDS OF CHICKEN, PORK, OR TOFU)**

10 dried guajillo chilies

7 dried mulato negro chilies

7 dried pasilla chilies

4 dried cascabel chilies

4 tablespoons avocado oil, divided

8 cloves garlic

1 small white onion, peeled and
   quartered

2 whole cloves

4 whole allspice berries

1 teaspoon anise

1 teaspoon ground Mexican cinnamon
   (canela)

1 teaspoon Mexican oregano

6 black peppercorns

1 yerba santa leaf

2 large plantains

2 dried apricots

1 ounce dark chocolate, melted

¼ cup raw almonds

¼ cup sesame seeds, toasted
    until golden

½ cup raisins

Toast all the chilies in a heavy cast-iron pan until the skins blister. Open all the windows while you are toasting and make sure you don't inhale the smoke. Stem, seed, and de-vein chilies, then soak them in 3 cups of very hot water until soft. Set aside both the chilies and the water for later. Heat 2 tablespoons of the oil, add garlic and onion, and cook for 3 to 5 minutes, until tender. Add the cloves, allspice berries, anise, cinnamon, oregano, and peppercorns into a spice mill and grind until very fine. Then, in small amounts, combine in a food processor the garlic and onion, chilies, yerba santa, plantains, apricots, chocolate, almonds, sesame seeds, and raisins, along with the ground spices. As you process, add a little of the water that held the soaked chilies until you have a very smooth paste.

Add the remaining avocado oil to a pan and add the paste, gently frying on all sides until it is dry and smooth, about 15 to 20 minutes. When it has cooled, refrigerate (or freeze) until needed. It can also be thinned with 2 cups of chicken broth when mixing with chicken, pork, (or even tofu).

---

### ⇶ *Jerk Spice Marinade* ⇷

This recipe celebrates allspice cuddled by other spices that enhance its flavor and action. Use this rub on chicken, shrimp, pork, or vegetables.

The term *jerk* refers to spice-rub culinary practice that evolved from cross-cultural contact. It was developed when Africans taken as slaves to the Caribbean came into contact with indigenous Arawak and Taíno peoples. Make this rub in advance for the best flavor.

**MAKES 1 TO 2 MARINATED MEALS FOR 4**

**DRY INGREDIENTS**

1 tablespoon ground allspice

1 tablespoon dried thyme leaves

1 teaspoon sea salt

1 teaspoon peppercorns

¼ stick cinnamon

1 teaspoon ground cayenne pepper
    (optional)

**WET INGREDIENTS**

1 clove garlic

1 thumb fresh ginger, peeled

2 tablespoons dark brown sugar

Grind the dry ingredients in a spice grinder and blend the wet ingredients in a blender. Combine the wet mixture with the dry and mix thoroughly with a spatula. Rub it on your meat or vegetables and let them marinate for a few hours in the fridge. Then roast them in the oven.

You can also prepare extra of the dried ingredients and store them separately in a cool, dry place, adding in the wet ingredients when needed for a future meal. If you have leftover wet ingredients, store them in a glass jar in the fridge for up to a month.

---

## AMCHOOR (*Mangifera*; *Mangifera indica*)

Amchoor is a spice powder made from dried, unripe mangoes and used as a citrusy seasoning to impart a sour, tangy fruit flavor to a meal without any added moisture. Amchoor is high in iron and vitamins A, C, and E and is used to improve digestion and reduce stomach acid and gastroesophageal reflex disease (GERD).

→ *Amchoor Turmeric Potatoes* ←

**SERVES 2**

1 teaspoon ground amchoor

1 teaspoon ground turmeric

¼ teaspoon ground cayenne pepper
   (optional)

¼ teaspoon ground cumin

½ teaspoon sea salt

2 tablespoons coconut oil or virgin
   cold-pressed olive oil

2 cups potatoes diced into
   1-inch cubes

½ cup coriander leaf

½ cup Greek yogurt

Combine all the spices and oil in a bowl and then stir in the potatoes and mix well. (If you do not eat potatoes you may use yucca as a substitute.) You can then fry or roast the potatoes. If frying, add a little more oil to the pan and cook over a medium heat until browned. Otherwise, place in an oiled roasting pan and roast at 400°F for 45 minutes. Top with fresh chopped coriander leaf and a little Greek yogurt.

---

## ANISE (*Pimpinella anisum*)

True anise is a dainty, aromatic annual (unrelated to star anise) from a flowering tree, that tastes and smells like licorice. Anise seed is a strong carminative, a remedy for flatulence, but it can be used to enhance overall digestion as well. It is also antimicrobial and antifungal, which makes it useful in treating candida infections.

A simple infusion of the pulverized and strained seeds will work well for gas pains. It has also deservedly maintained a reputation for being an effective expectorant and antispasmodic, making it a respiratory herb. Using a chest rub made from the seeds or inhaling the essential oil soothes the bronchial passages and chest-related congestion.

Anise seeds contain estragole, phenylpropene, and anethole compounds that contribute to the tingly sensations in your mouth when you eat a handful of seeds. Anethole has been observed to exhibit estrogenic effects, which is probably why anise is used as a libido stimulant. It may also explain why an Iranian formula of 500 milligrams of anise, saffron, and celery seeds 3 times a day is beneficial for painful menstruations. Apply a strong decoction of the seeds to painful, swollen breasts or to stimulate the flow of milk in nursing mothers.

### ⇉ Anise for Gas ⇇

Grind 1 tablespoon of the seeds, simmer in a cup of hot water for 5 minutes, strain, and drink for gas pains or to reduce spasms.

### ⇉ Anise Chest Rub ⇇

Grind 3 tablespoons of seeds into a fine powder and add equal amounts of ground flaxseed. Make into a paste and apply warm to the chest during recovery from a chronic cough or bronchitis. Using the paste or inhaling the essential oil will soothe the bronchial passages and chest-related congestion.

### ⇉ Anise Liqueur ⇇

Mrs. Maud Grieve, an early twentieth-century British herbalist, suggested taking an anise liqueur in hot water as an immediate palliative for congested bronchial tubes, spasmodic asthma, and bronchitis.

In a pinch, buy a bottle of Greek ouzo or French anisette or arak, add a tablespoon of one of these liqueurs to a cup of hot water, and take 3 times a day to help soothe a chest cold.

## BARBERRY (*Berberis vulgaris*)

The dried berry of the common barberry plant is a common addition to Afghani, Persian, and Indian cuisines. The berries have a sharp and sour taste, providing a balance to spicy dishes. They are used in Iranian wedding foods because their sourness represents the idea that marriage is not always sweet and rosy. Barberries are added to rice pilafs, curries, and chutneys and are used as a flavoring for poultry. Jams, preserves, and jellies are also made with these berries.

The barberry contains berberine, a natural anti-inflammatory that balances the immune system and is antibacterial. Berberine supplements are widely used to reduce blood glucose levels in diabetes or prediabetes and as a remedy for food poisoning and diarrhea. The berries are rich in vitamin C.

## BASIL, ITALIAN (*Ocimum basilicum*)

Basil, the "king of herbs," is a potent aromatic herb that awakens any food it touches. It is an antihistamine, antibacterial, and anti-inflammatory, and is rich in beta-carotene (an antioxidant good for the lungs and eyes) and vitamin K. It is easy to grow during the summer heat and can be generously added to salads, where it mixes well with tomatoes and feta cheese. Here are three different approaches to using basil as both food and medicine.

### → *Basil Apple Juice for Sinus Congestion* ←

One of my early mentors was Dr. Mary Raugust, a pediatrician, psychologist, mother of six, and an herbalist who was the first woman dean of Harvard Medical School. She was a feminist who believed in caring for oneself and one's children with as little medical intervention as possible. She fought against quotas of women in medicine and was an early proponent of herbal medicine for women and their families. One day when I had to travel and had a lot of sinus congestion and ear pain, she made me this very simple but effective basil recipe, so I could actually get on the plane and fly.

**MAKES 1 SERVING**

2 to 3 large organic apples          ½ cup fresh basil leaves

Juice the apples to yield about 8 ounces of juice. Add the juice to a blender along with the basil leaves and blend well. Drink 8 ounces twice a day to ease sinus congestion. The juice should be made fresh each time before use for greatest benefit.

## → *Basil Pesto* ←

Basil pesto is a tasty medicinal food that I like to make in big batches a few times a year. It is one of the best ways to always have basil on hand, as a food and medicine. Spring and summer are the best times to collect fresh basil and gather friends and family in the kitchen to make pesto that will last for several months in the freezer. Basil and garlic are antibacterial and antioxidant, and the olive oil and pine nuts nourish the brain and joints. Usually one adds cheese, but it's possible to make pesto without the Romano or Parmesan cheese, and it also freezes better without it.

**MAKES 7 CUPS (ENOUGH FOR 4 MEALS, SERVING 4)**

4 cups densely packed fresh basil leaves

1 cup pine nuts

6 garlic cloves, minced

1 cup virgin cold-pressed olive oil

Sea salt

Freshly ground black pepper

1 cup freshly grated Parmigiano-Reggiano cheese (optional)

Put the fresh basil leaves and pine nuts in a food processor and pulse several times. Add the garlic and pulse, slowly adding the olive oil in a steady stream so that it emulsifies. Add salt and pepper to taste. Blend grated cheese in at the end, if using.

Divide up basil portions into small freezer-friendly containers of about 4 ounces each and freeze until you need the pesto for a quick meal. It goes well over noodles, vegetables, shrimp, tofu, or beef, or it can be added to an omelet.

## → *Topical Basil for Arthritis Anti-inflammatory* ←

One of the herbalists I worked with in Mexico demonstrated a simple anti-inflammatory recipe for swollen or arthritic joints.

Grind fresh basil in a molcajete or chop it in a blender, add a little fresh leaf lard (if you do not have lard on hand you may substitute coconut oil), and make a paste. Apply the paste to the painful joint and wrap the joint in a cloth for several hours or overnight. In the morning, wash it off with sea salt, rub dry, and apply *mota* (see "Herbal Liniment" on page 22) for use during an active day. Do this for 3 days or for as long as needed.

**BERBERE**

The word *berbere* is Amharic for "pepper." Berbere is an ancient Ethiopian spice mix that includes chili peppers, garlic, basil, korarima, rue, ajwain or radhuni, nigella, and fenugreek. A simple berbere recipe with easy-to-source ingredients includes ground ginger, ground red pepper, ground cloves, and ground cinnamon. There is no universal recipe for berbere, but chili peppers and fenugreek are consistent. Berbere is used in an Ethiopian sauce called *awaze*, often used to braise meats. It is also used as a base for traditional Ethiopian dishes like *doro wot* (chicken stew) and *misir wot* (lentil stew). The spice mix is rich in vitamins, minerals, and soluble fiber.

## ⇝ *Misir Wot* ⇜

I have adapted this recipe from the version made by the Oaktown Spice Shop in Oakland.

**SERVES 2 TO 4**

4 tablespoons ghee or unsalted butter

1 medium yellow onion, finely chopped

4 cloves garlic, finely chopped

1 cup small red lentils, rinsed and drained

1 large tomato, chopped

2 tablespoons berbere, divided

4 cups water or fresh chicken broth

Sea salt

Heat the ghee in a saucepan over medium heat. Add the onions and cook until tender, about 10 minutes. Add the garlic and cook for a minute. Add the lentils, tomato, 1 tablespoon of the berbere, and the water or chicken broth to the pan. Bring to a simmer.

Reduce heat to medium-low and simmer, stirring occasionally, until the lentils are tender, about 45 minutes. Stir in the remaining tablespoon of the berbere and season generously with sea salt.

## BLACK CUMIN SEEDS (*Nigella sativa*)

The *Nigella sativa* plant, also referred to as black cumin, is a different species from cumin. Black cumin seeds were used in ancient Egypt, and they are used worldwide as food and medicine. Black cumin seed oil is considered a curative for over a hundred diseases in Islamic medicine. The Muslim prophet Mohammed said that black cumin seed is a cure for every disease, except death. The main constituents in the black cumin seed responsible for its medicinal properties are thymoquinone and alpha-hederin. The seeds have been well studied for their benefits to the heart as an anti-inflammatory, and they are used as part of the pancreatic cancer protocol as an anticancer remedy. It has also been shown to have antidepressant, anxiolytic, and memory-enhancing effects. Research suggests that black cumin seed oil aids weight loss and reduction of nonalcoholic fatty liver disease in women.

## ⇒ *Black Cumin Seed Oil Salad Dressing* ⇐

Black cumin seed oil is an effective way to incorporate the seed into your diet.

**MAKES 3 CUPS**

1 cup virgin cold-pressed olive oil

1 teaspoon black cumin seed oil

2 cups apple cider vinegar

1 clove garlic, crushed

Sea salt

Mix all ingredients together and use a few tablespoons over cold lettuce and bitter greens, topped with feta cheese. Store in a glass bottle in the fridge for up to 2 weeks.

---

### CARAWAY (*Carum carvi*)

I grew up eating rye bread with caraway seeds, and whenever I eat that stick-in-your-teeth seed I am transported back to the deli and eating a corned beef on rye and with my grandpa Charlie. These days, I rarely get to a deli, but I love to add caraway to biscuits, coleslaw, and steamed cabbage. Caraway is a quick remedy for flatulence, heartburn, and acid reflux, so the next time you experience indigestion or gas chew on a few of the raw seeds. I keep a little bowl of caraway and fennel seeds on the dinner table to remind me that caraway seeds, like dill and mint, are rich in the volatile oil carvone, which gives the seeds their carminative properties. An infusion of the seeds can be used to treat bronchitis, colds, coughs, and a sore throat, and an essential oil made from the seeds can be used in cough remedies, particularly for children. The seed also contains a mild antihistamine and has antimicrobial properties, and caraway oil is used as an emmenagogue to relieve menstrual cramping. Topically caraway can be used in mouthwashes and skin rubs to improve blood flow. When a child has a cough or cold, grind caraway seed into a powder, add them to oil of lavender, and rub on the chest and temples to help them fall asleep.

### CARDAMOM (*Elettaria cardamomum*)

Native to the Indian subcontinent, cardamom is a popular cooking and baking spice. It is an aromatic, resinous seed, rich in essential oils. It is the third most expensive spice in the world. As an aromatic, it is a perfect antispasmodic and carminative. It is a handy kitchen spice for stomach cramps, indigestion, and inflammatory bowel syndrome, and it is used for relieving nausea and clearing congestion from colds, flus, and allergies. It is also mildly sedative, as it contains the phytochemical cineole, which is responsible for calming nerves, clearing the head, and killing bacteria that cause bad breath.

⇒ *Cardamom Saffron Coffee* ⇐

**MAKES 1 SERVING**

This is an adaptation of a popular Middle Eastern recipe. It's rich in mood-boosting ingredients. Add 3 green cardamom pods and 2 cloves of saffron to your coffee beans when you grind them. Then prepare the coffee as a drip or in a French press. Gently heat cream or almond milk in a saucepan and add a few stigmas of saffron to the milk. Froth it and pour the coffee and milk together.

**CAYENNE (*Capsicum annuum*)**

Cayenne is a popular spice in culinary dishes, particularly in the Americas. It is a powerful rubefacient and vasodilator. It is considered one of the most potent stimulants in the plant world, so when you consider well-being that requires stimulation, consider cayenne pepper. The capsaicin in cayenne allows blood to move freely through the body, giving cayenne its warming qualities. It is excellent for people who tend to get cold easily. The capsaicin is also responsible for thinning mucus, which is especially useful for chest and nasal congestion. Cayenne stimulates the hypothalamus (a stress response center in the body) and thereby can cool down the body. Topically, cayenne is used for painful muscle spasms, sprains, and pleurisy.

Capsaicin can be purchased as a cream over the counter or may be found in higher doses of prescription creams compounded by pharmacies for those experiencing intense pain from fibromyalgia or neuropathy.

⇒ *Hot Cayenne Cocoa* ⇐

**MAKES 1 TO 2 SERVINGS**

Who can turn away from a delicious drink that warms, and then warms again? Cayenne and chocolate are kissing cousins. Both indigenous to Mexico, they complement each other in surprising ways. This recipe is a good food for your heart, brain, and spirits.

Add 1 tablespoon of raw local honey or 10 drops of stevia to 2 cups of milk or coconut or hemp milk, or any mixture you prefer. Warm the milk in a saucepan and stir in 2 heaping tablespoons of sugar-free cocoa powder with a wire whisk. Take off the heat and add a pinch of ground cayenne pepper to warm the cockles of your heart.

---

## → *Chocolate Cayenne Coconut Joy* ←

My husband, Rudolph, created this chocolate cayenne coconut joy candy. Making this requires a few hours in the afternoon, so gather kids and elders alike on a weekend and make a pile of healthy candy for everyone to take home. This recipe makes plenty of candy that can be frozen for future use.

**MAKES 24 CANDIES**

½ cup dark agave, raw local honey, or maple syrup; or 20 to 25 drops liquid stevia

2 tablespoons butter

2 cups unsweetened shredded coconut, lightly packed

¼ to ¾ teaspoon ground cayenne pepper, depending on your taste

17 ounces dark chocolate (no sugar added), chopped or broken into small pieces

30 to 35 lightly roasted and unsalted almonds

In a saucepan, bring the agave to a low boil over medium heat. Add the butter and melt it, stirring occasionally. Once fully integrated, remove from heat and let sit for 2 to 3 minutes. Add the coconut slowly, stirring until it is fully coated. Then add the cayenne. Note: when making the candy with children in mind, set aside some of the mixture before adding the cayenne in case the kids don't like the "heat."

Put a sheet of parchment paper on a clean cutting board. Pour the agave coconut mixture onto the parchment paper, spreading it with a spatula or the flat side of a knife. Spread the mixture to about a ½-inch thickness. Form into a 9 x 4-inch rectangle and cover with another piece of parchment paper. Using a rolling pin or bottle, lightly roll the mixture outward until it is about ¼ inch thick. Allow the mixture to cool slightly, remove the top parchment, then cut the mixture into strips about 1 inch wide. Working crosswise cut the strips again into 2-inch rectangles. (Tip: Coat your knife with butter to keep the mixture from sticking.) Slide the coconut squares, still on their parchment, onto a half-sheet pan, allowing them to set in the refrigerator while you prepare the chocolate.

Next, create a double boiler for the chocolate. Put the chocolate into a heat-proof bowl. Set the bowl over a pan of simmering water but don't allow the bowl to touch the water. Melt the chocolate, stirring constantly with a rubber spatula, until it is smooth. Remove the melted chocolate from the heat.

Place another piece of parchment paper on the cutting board. Working quickly while the chocolate is still warm, spread a thin layer of the chocolate into a rectangle that is more or less the size of the sheet of coconut squares, using only half of the melted chocolate. When finished, place it in the refrigerator to cool for 15 minutes or until firm. Remove the coconut squares and chocolate from the refrigerator and immediately turn out the coconut squares on top of the chocolate. Press down firmly using your hands. Remove the parchment from the coconut. Using a knife, separate the coconut and chocolate squares following the cuts made earlier.

Top each coconut square with a roasted almond. Using a spoon, ladle the rest of the melted chocolate across the coconut squares, creating an even layer. Refrigerate the pan for 20 to 30 minutes to allow the chocolate to harden. Recut the squares and refrigerate until ready to serve.

---

### CELERY (*Apium graveolens*)

The oft-ignored celery provides every part of her plant for food and medicine. The root and stalk can be used as an effective diuretic, and the seeds are harvested as a flavoring spice or for their essential oil and can be used whole or ground and mixed with sea salt to make celery salt. The use of celery seeds dates to 4000 BCE when ancient Greeks used them for pain, and the Romans used them as an aphrodisiac. In Ayurvedic medicine, celery seeds are used to treat gout and arthritis. The aromatic seed is also a bitter digestive and liver stimulant and, taken as a tea or smoothie at night, can be deeply relaxing and encourage sleep.

### CHAMOMILE (*Matricaria chamomilla; Chamaemelum nobile*)

German chamomile and Roman chamomile are similar-looking species, and while both are used medicinally, German chamomile is considered to be the more medicinally potent. Chamomile is commonly used as a soothing sedative and as a gastrointestinal aid. It is a carminative, antispasmodic, anti-inflammatory, antibacterial, antifungal, and antiseptic, and it is used for indigestion, bloating, heartburn, flatulence, and diarrhea. A flavonoid in the flower heads called apigenin binds to benzodiazepine receptor sites, making the plant a mild but effective nervous system depressant. A volatile oil in the plant called azulene, which turns blue when it is distilled, is a strong anti-inflammatory, combating fever and relieving stomach tension. The plant is also very effective externally for a variety of skin problems, such as eczema or psoriasis, and chamomile ointment is equal or superior to hydrocortisone as an anti-inflammatory agent. A strong infusion of the flower head is effective for its medicinal qualities; a weak infusion functions as a general tonic. Chamomile is very gentle and can be used with children who have stomachaches or are anxious.

### ↠ Slumber Smoothie ↞

The chamomile tea and cherries in this recipe will help induce sleep, while the mangoes, seeds, and coconut will support blood sugar throughout the night so you can rest peacefully. Blueberries or frozen bananas make a good substitute for mangoes. Drink this smoothie an hour before you want to go to sleep.

**MAKES 3 SERVINGS**

1 cup almond or coconut milk

½ cup strong cold chamomile tea

1 cup frozen (or fresh) cherries

1 cup frozen mangoes or blueberries

1 teaspoon flaxseeds (or flaxseed oil or lemon-flavored fish oil)

½ teaspoon chia seeds

1 tablespoon coconut cream or coconut oil

3 to 7 drops liquid stevia

1 drop vanilla extract (optional)

Combine all ingredients in the blender and blend until smooth. Keep a quart of strong chamomile tea in the fridge or make Chamomile Tea Ice Cubes to add to evening smoothies. Drink this smoothie as often as you like.

### CILANTRO, CORIANDER (*Coriandrum sativum*)

Cilantro is a hearty, annual plant, similar to parsley, that is sometimes referred to as Chinese parsley. All parts of the plant are edible; however, the leaves and seeds are most popularly used in cuisine. The leaves of the plant are especially rich in vitamins A, C, and K. The aldehyde molecule in the plant gives cilantro its particularly strong aroma and taste. You either love it or you hate it. This is because some people have a genetic variation that causes them to perceive the aldehydes in cilantro as tasting like soap, hence, the strong aversion. Cilantro is widely regarded as a plant that helps eliminate heavy metals from the body; thus the leaves of the plant are typically eaten fresh, as a garnish or flavoring.

Coriander, the seed of the cilantro plant, is typically dried and is more medicinally potent than the leaves. An infusion of the seeds is an excellent remedy for upper abdominal complaints, flatulence, and mild cramps related to gastrointestinal upset. It is also an effective carminative. The volatile oil, linalool, is the same oil found in lavender, bergamot, citrus, and orange flowers. The oils in the seeds are found to have strong antimicrobial and antibacterial properties.

## ↠ *Coriander Pesto* ↞

This is a healthy and delicious pesto that can be used on pasta, rice, or tofu or as a dipping sauce for vegetables. Double the recipe and freeze it in small containers, so it can be pulled out for a quick healthy meal.

**MAKES 5 CUPS (ENOUGH FOR 6 TO 8 MEALS FOR 4)**

3 cups firmly packed fresh cilantro leaves and stems

1 cup firmly packed Italian, flat leaf parsley leaves and stems

½ cup chopped raw pine nuts (or raw walnuts)

¼ teaspoon sea salt

2 cloves garlic

½ to ¾ cup virgin cold-pressed olive oil

Using a food processor, place ¼ of each of the ingredients in the bowl and add olive oil in slowly as you blend. Keep adding ingredients until they are all blended and smooth.

## ↠ *Tummy Bloat Tea* ↞

**MAKES ½ CUP, ABOUT 8 SERVINGS**

Combine 1 ounce each of the seeds of coriander, anise, caraway, and fennel and store in an amber glass jar in the dark. When you need help in digesting a heavy meal or a meal that has caused gas, simmer a heaping tablespoon of the seed mixture in 2 cups of water for 15 minutes and drink. For children, add a touch of raw local honey.

## CINNAMON (*Cinnamomum verum*)

The cinnamon that is stocked in supermarkets is dried bark from the young branches and shoots from the cinnamon tree, a small evergreen. There are two varieties:

Ceylon and cassia. Cassia is native to southern China and the one most commonly found in supermarkets. Ceylon or "true cinnamon" is native to South India and Sri Lanka. Common cinnamon originates from Sri Lanka and is the variety known as canela, or Mexican cinnamon. Traditional Chinese herbalists prescribe cinnamon to circulate vital energy through the abdomen and to treat chills, influenza, and parasites. Added to well-cooked rice, cinnamon is an excellent remedy for diarrhea.

Cinnamon is widely used to treat various digestive disorders as well. It can stimulate appetite, reduce stomach acid, and strengthen the gut wall. It is also used in the treatment of colds, flus, and coughs and is known to increase the blood flow to the hands and feet.

Methylhydroxychalcone, a polyphenol compound in cassia cinnamon, lowers triglycerides and blood sugar, so cinnamon can be beneficial for people with diabetes. Cinnamon's antibacterial and antifungal qualities make it useful for treating Candida albicans and Helicobacter pylori, the cause of stomach ulcers.

Cinnamon can be taken as an infusion, decoction, tincture, essential oil, or just ground and put on food as a seasoning. Cinnamon oil is a natural pesticide that also repels mosquitos.

CAUTION: Cinnamon is a uterine stimulant and should be avoided in large quantities during pregnancy.

## → *Cinnamon Tea* ←

**MAKES 1 SERVING**

I love the smell of cinnamon, as it is deeply relaxing to the nervous system. There are so many ways to use cinnamon in foods, teas, and baked goods. Cinnamon tea has long been used as a breakfast tea in Mexico, where cinnamon is also added to coffee.

Simmer half a stick of cinnamon in 1½ cups of boiling water for 10 minutes, until the water browns. Strain and drink.

## → *Cinnamon Turmeric Butter Coffee* ←

**MAKES 1 SERVING**

1 cup strong coffee

½ teaspoon ground cinnamon

½ teaspoon ground turmeric

Dash of freshly ground black pepper

1 teaspoon raw butter or ghee

Cream or coconut or hemp milk to taste

To the cup of coffee, add all the ingredients and warm but don't boil it. Blend together with a milk frother and enjoy as a morning drink.

---

### CLOVE (*Syzygium aromaticum*)

Cloves are the buds of an evergreen tree, picked and dried before they bloom. They are highly aromatic, warming stimulants, which makes them excellent digestive aids. They are also very strong germicides and antiseptics, useful in protecting against intestinal parasites. Eugenol, the active compound in cloves, kills bacteria and fungi. Clove oil is essentially pure eugenol and is found in many mouthwashes and toothpaste formulas. The oil is used to deaden the pain of a toothache and destroy bacteria in the mouth and can be applied topically for headaches, colds, arthritis, and muscle aches. A tea of the buds is appropriate for internal parasites, stomachaches, chills, vomiting, and nausea. Sucking on a few cloves makes an inexpensive breath freshener.

### CUMIN (*Cuminum cyminum*)

The dried seed of cumin, a member of the parsley family, is earthy, warm, and aromatic and is used in many cuisines. It is added to curries, chili powders, achiote blends, garam masala, adobos, *sofritos, bahaarat,* pickles, pastries, stews, soups, and cheese. The world's oldest culinary recipes include cumin—ancient Mesopotamian tablets show that cumin was used together with garlic and onion. The major essential oil in cumin is cuminaldehyde, which has analgesic, antidiabetic, anti-inflammatory, antibacterial, and estrogenic effects. Cumin is a stimulant, carminative, and astringent. In Ayurveda, it is widely used because it balances the three doshas, or life energies, of vata, pitta, and kapha. It is often toasted to top yogurt or may be sautéed in ghee and added to lentils to help relax the muscles and the nervous system. Cumin, called *comino* in Spanish, is a staple of Mexican food, often seasoning beans and taco fillings.

### ↠ *Garam Masala* ↞

This recipe celebrates cumin as one of our most delectable healing spices. Garam masala is the Indian spice mixture that joins medicine with flavor in a mix that always excites. Ayurvedic medicine uses this mixture to heat the body and accelerate metabolism and energy. There are many ways to make a garam masala mix, but I love to start with whole seeds and make it from scratch—it's easy and worth the effort.

**MAKES ABOUT ½ CUP**

3 tablespoons coriander seeds

2 bay leaves

2 tablespoons cumin seeds

2 tablespoons black peppercorns

1 teaspoon whole cloves

1 teaspoon freshly grated nutmeg

1 teaspoon fennel seed

1 whole cinnamon stick

½ teaspoon ground cayenne pepper

2 tablespoons cardamom pods

Add all the ingredients except the cardamom pods to a large sauté pan and toast, stirring over low heat for about 10 minutes until the seeds are slightly browned. Set aside and let cool and then place them, along with the cardamom pods, in a spice blender. Blend to a medium-fine grind and store in an amber glass jar in a dark cabinet. You may use this mixture with a variety of dishes, by adding it at the start of cooking curries, vegetables, or lamb, chicken, or fish stews or sprinkle in bread or muffins.

---

## DILL (*Anethum graveolens*)

Dill seeds and leaves are used for medicine and food across many different cultures. Dill seed contains dillanoside, coumarins, volatile oils, flavonoids, and phenolic acids. A remedy for flatulence and indigestion, dill is also an adaptogen and a nervine. Dill water or "gripe water" is an ancient remedy for a colicky baby.

Use dill on salad, yogurt, coleslaw, potatoes, pickles, beans, and frittatas. Dill seeds and leaves go everywhere on most everything.

### → *Homemade Dill Mayonnaise* ←

Once you taste your own homemade mayonnaise you will never go back to commercial varieties. Most store-bought mayonnaise uses soy or canola oils, not the best oils for health. Use either avocado oil for its mild taste or olive oil, which will give the stronger taste of olives to this delicate recipe. Note: make sure you know the source of your eggs to ensure they are good quality.

**MAKES 1 CUP**

1 large free-range egg yolk

1½ teaspoons fresh lemon juice

1 teaspoon white wine vinegar

¼ teaspoon mustard (optional)

½ teaspoon sea salt

1 cup avocado oil or virgin cold-pressed olive oil

1 teaspoon dill leaf

All ingredients should be at room temperature. Whisk together all the ingredients except the oil and the dill until smooth. Put in a blender and at medium speed slowly drizzle oil in a little at a time, blending evenly until the mixture thickens. This may take 5 to 10 minutes. Then add in the dill leaf and stir by hand. Put the mayonnaise in a glass jar and store in the fridge for up to 2 weeks.

---

### EPAZOTE (*Dysphania ambrosioides*)

The word *epazote* comes from the Nahuatl words for skunk (*epatl*) and sweat (*tzotl*) because of its stinky smell, though it tastes delicious. It's found in most kitchen gardens in Mexico as well as in farmers markets and Mexican stores in the United States. It's a staple herb of Mexican cuisine that seasons black beans, quesadillas, tamales, chilaquiles, and enchiladas. Epazote is part of the goosefoot family of plants, which also includes quinoa (*Chenopodium quinoa*), quelites (*Amaranthus polygonoides*), and huauzontle (*Chenopodium nuttalliae*) with their characteristic tight green edible buds. Epazote contains oil of chenopodium and ascaridole, both of which are effective anthelmintics; hence its other name, "wormseed." Drink a tea of dried epazote for 10 days to expel intestinal worms.

> → *Grilled Cheese and Epazote* ←

Epazote and cheese are a perfect match; the pungent flavor of epazote is balanced by the rich, creamy, subtle flavor of a grilling cheese. A simple one is to make a grilled cheese sandwich with your favorite cheese and a few epazote leaves and sliced tomatoes. If you don't want to use bread, you can put a grillable cheese like a panela, paneer, or a Greek cheese like saganaki in a small frying pan and place thinly sliced tomatoes and epazote leaves atop and cover while it all melts together.

---

### FENNEL (*Foeniculum vulgare*)

Fennel is a rich source of potassium, fiber, and iron, making it useful for treating anemia, regulating cholesterol, and maintaining healthy blood pressure. Fennel seeds have traditionally been used as digestive tonics, acting as carminatives, laxatives, and digestive stimulants and relieving anxiety-related digestive problems. They also help to regulate menstruation, reduce PMS, and allay menopausal symptoms. The aroma of fennel essential oil helps lift one's mood. The fennel plant can be steamed and the seed can be incorporated into a tea, or just chewed after eating.

## → *Tomatoes, Panela Cheese, and Fennel Pollen* ←

**SERVES 2 TO 4**

Fennel pollen is gathered from the flowers of fennel and delivers a potent and powerful wake-up call to your taste buds. It goes with many foods, but I like to keep it simple and enjoy it with the well-defined and simple flavors of tomato and cheese.

Panela is a cheese made in Mexico that you can purchase in the United States. Its texture is similar to that of Greek kasseri cheese and to Indian paneer, both of which make good substitutes. You may also use a plain goat cheese.

Place 4 ounces of cheese in a small baking dish, cover with a tomato slice, drizzle with virgin cold-pressed olive oil, and sprinkle on a pinch of fennel pollen. Bake for 5 to 7 minutes at 350°F, or until it is soft and warm.

## GINGER (*Zingiber officinale*)

Ginger is an all-around panacea and the fresh root, powder, and candy are all essential ingredients to have in your herbal medicine cabinet. Ginger reduces nausea, vomiting, inflammation, and the frequency of colds, and lowers cholesterol and improves metabolism. Fresh root should always be available in the kitchen. Adding a little fresh grated ginger to orange juice makes a healing drink for the liver, and it's an easy-to-take anti-inflammatory and spicy addition to any dish. Ginger adds heat to food without burning the way a chili might, and it's a major ingredient of Bengali curry, which is always worthwhile spending an afternoon to make.

## → *Candied Ginger, Mango, and Blueberries* ←

There are so many wonderful ways to use fresh and powdered ginger. This is a refreshing favorite which uses candied ginger for a summer party.

**SERVES 8**

4 mangoes, cubed

4 cups fresh blueberries

1 cup candied ginger, finely sliced

Juice of 4 limes

Mix the mango, blueberries, and ginger together and toss with fresh lime juice.

## HORSERADISH (*Armoracia rusticana*)

The root of this plant, a member of the Brassicaceae family, is often prepared by cutting or grating the tuber and immediately preserving it in vinegar or citric acid. Horseradish contains mustard oil and allyl isothiocyanate, volatile oils that are released when the root is cut. Horseradish is a stimulant, laxative, rubefacient, diuretic, and antiseptic. It is a particularly good food to add with fatty and/or oily meals, stimulating the digestive system for better absorption. When used externally, horseradish is a powerful rubefacient, making it helpful for musculoskeletal conditions. It is beneficial for urinary tract infections (UTIs), acute bronchitis, colds, sore throats, and sinusitis. Horseradish is a common addition to a Seder dinner on Passover, shared as a bitter vegetable, a symbol of the bitterness of slavery.

### →» *Horseradish Vinegar or Honey* «←

Horseradish is a central ingredient in the *Caliente Curación* recipe on page 48; however, if you need help in a pinch, horseradish vinegar or horseradish honey will do.

Finely grate a freshly peeled horseradish root and add ½ teaspoon of horseradish per cup of raw local honey. Let it sit for several hours. Take a teaspoon every 4 hours. Don't ingest more than this recommended dose as it can upset your stomach.

## LEMONGRASS (*Cymbopogon*; *Cymbopogon citratus*)

Lemongrass is a cooling herb beneficial for indigestion, bloating, or constipation. It is rich in minerals such as potassium, zinc, iron, and magnesium and is a good source of vitamins B and C. The citral in lemongrass is a strong antimicrobial, antifungal, and anti-inflammatory and is beneficial for arthritis. Eating or drinking lemongrass or even inhaling its aroma reduces stress, headaches, and anxiety. Planting lemongrass in your garden reduces mosquitoes. Lemongrass root can be purchased fresh or kept frozen for use in coconut curried vegetables, for hot tea, or to make the Spicy Lemongrass Ginger Ale (recipe follows), which helps to relieve symptoms of laryngitis, sore throats, and bronchitis.

CAUTION: Avoid lemongrass during pregnancy. Two constituents of lemongrass, citral and myrcene, have been shown to have adverse effects in pregnancy in animal research. In high doses, myrcene can cause abnormalities in the skeletal development of a fetus or miscarriage.

## → *Spicy Lemongrass Ginger Ale* ←

**SERVES 8**

1 pound fresh ginger, peeled and
    chopped

3 lemongrass roots each about 4 inches
    long, chopped

½ small serrano chili, seeds removed
    (optional)

½ cup raw local honey

4 cups water

Juice of ½ lime

Sparkling mineral water

Blend the ginger, lemongrass, and chili, if using, in a blender and process until pureed. Pour the puree into a saucepan and add the honey and water. Bring to a boil and then simmer for 10 minutes. Cool, and strain into a glass jar. Chill in the refrigerator. When ready to use, add ½ cup of the syrup and the lime juice to a glass full of ice and sparkling mineral water and serve.

---

### MARJORAM (*Origanum majorana*)

Marjoram is used for cooking and medicine alike. It is similar to its cousin, basil, but it has a sweeter flavor. Marjoram relaxes the nervous system without causing drowsiness and relieves stress and anxiety. Rich in volatile oils, it is a tonic for lungs, as well as an expectorant.

Well known as a seasoning herb, marjoram and marjoram oil can be used to treat a lack of appetite, poor digestion, gastritis, and ulcers, and as a tea it is helpful for food poisoning. Inhaling the vapor of the essential oil is calming and lowers blood pressure. Marjoram balances the menstrual cycle and is also an emmenagogue and galactagogue. Fresh marjoram has a subtle yet deep minty flavor and makes a wonderful addition to a chicken or pea soup.

### MUSTARD SEED (*Brassica juncea*; *Brassica nigra*; *Sinapis alba*)

The seeds of the mustard plant are typically ground and mixed with water and vinegar to create a condiment. Toasted mustard seeds are widely used in Indian cooking. Rich in selenium and magnesium, the seeds are anti-inflammatory. Ground mustard seed poultices can be applied for neuralgia, sciatica, gout, and pneumonia. Its pungent and warming qualities also make it effective for skin infections. Mustard seeds are used in recovery from cancer, diabetes, cardiovascular disease, and neuropathic pain.

## OREGANO (*Origanum vulgare*)

Greek oregano regulates and alleviates irregular and painful menstruation and reduces vasomotor symptoms in menopause making it helpful for women of all ages. When concentrated as an oil it is a powerful antibacterial, antifungal, and immune-system enhancer. Oil of oregano helps reduce the symptoms of colds and small intestinal bacterial overgrowth. The fresh plant can be used daily, but the oil in capsules should be used no more than 10 days out of the month, followed by probiotic-enriching foods.

## OREGANO, MEXICAN (*Lippia graveolens*)

Mexican oregano is a member of the verbena family and is used to add a little citrus flavor to food. It has a flavor similar to oregano, and it is rich in thymol, which gives it its antiseptic qualities.

## PAPRIKA (*Capsicum annuum*)

Paprika is the ground spice of the different varieties of the *Capsicum annuum* species, usually the bell pepper or the tomato pepper. Paprika can range from mild to hot: sweet paprika is crushed pepper with half the seeds removed, and hot paprika is crushed pepper with all parts of the pepper used. Paprika is used in cooking to flavor and color rice, stews, soups, and meats. It is a popular spice used in Hungarian, Mexican, Portuguese, and Creole cooking. Paprika is an antioxidant and lowers blood glucose levels.

### ⇻ *Shakshouka* ⇇

This is a quick and easy recipe to make for any meal of the day, and yet it provides complex flavors worthy of brunch festivities. Building on the foundation of smoked paprika, shakshouka originated in Tunisia and is now enjoyed the world over. I have adapted it a bit to add additional medicinal spices. It's similar to the Mexican dish chilaquiles though instead of an oregano red sauce, it emphasizes a paprika and cumin flavored profile.

**SERVES 4 TO 6**

4 tablespoons virgin cold-pressed olive oil

1 small onion, finely chopped

1 clove garlic, finely chopped

1 red bell pepper

Two 14.5-ounce cans chopped tomatoes

4 Roma tomatoes, diced

2 teaspoons ground smoked paprika

2 teaspoons ground coriander

½ teaspoon ground cardamom

½ teaspoon caraway seeds

½ teaspoon sea salt

½ teaspoon freshly ground black pepper

Pinch of ground cayenne pepper
 (optional)

4 to 6 free-range eggs

Feta cheese (optional)

Fresh cilantro or parsley, chopped

In a deep sauté pan over medium heat, add the olive oil and sauté the onion, garlic, and bell pepper. When the onions are translucent, add all the tomatoes, stir, and then add all the spices and let simmer on low heat for 30 minutes. Make small indentations in the sauce for each egg and then gently pour an egg into each one. Sprinkle with feta cheese, if using, cover, and cook for 5 minutes on low or until the eggs are fully cooked. When you are ready to serve, add 1 or 2 eggs to a plate with plenty of sauce and top with fresh cilantro or parsley.

---

### ROSEMARY (*Rosmarinus officinalis*)

Rosemary has historically been used for a variety of ailments, including respiratory and circulatory complaints, liver congestion, digestive disorders, and anxiety. It can be used internally for indigestion, to prevent thrombosis, and to increase menstrual production and urine flow and externally for rheumatoid arthritis and circulatory problems. Topically, rosemary is used to activate hair growth and treat dandruff or oily scalp, eczema, and psoriasis. Essential oil of rosemary is beneficial for concentration and memory. I explore rosemary further in chapter 8.

### SAFFRON (*Crocus sativus*)

The threads of the *Crocus sativus* plant provide the exotic spice we call saffron. The pistils contain volatile oils and compounds responsible for imbuing the herb with antioxidant, antidepressant, and anticancer properties. Safranal and crocin are compounds that give saffron its distinct color and flavor, its medicinal qualities, and its high mineral and vitamin content. Saffron is well established as an antidepressant. In traditional medicine, saffron is used as a carminative, antispasmodic, and diaphoretic. An easy way to include saffron in your diet is to add it to rice and vegetables or make a tea by adding several threads to a ginger and honey tea.

### SAVORY (*Satureja hortensis*)

Savory includes several species of the *Satureja* genus and is typically used as a spice or tea. Summer savory and winter savory are two species commonly used in food and medicine. Winter savory can be made into an antiseptic, carminative, and digestive tonic and is used in the treatment of bronchial congestion, nausea, diarrhea, and menstrual pain. Externally, a poultice of winter savory can be used to treat insect bites and bee stings. Summer savory is used in the treatment of low blood pressure.

### SEA SALT

Sea salt is often combined with herbs to enhance flavors in foods and to enhance the cleansing and restorative effects of herbs in salt baths. Unrefined sea salt has over ninety trace minerals that support bone health, digestion, and good sleep. Craving salt may be a sign of adrenal fatigue, and sea salt is especially good to combine with herbs when you experience fatigue and exhaustion as it enhances adrenal function.

### STAR ANISE, CHINESE (*Illicium verum*)

Star anise, unrelated to the anise plant, contains a chemical compound called shikimic acid that can be synthesized into an anti-influenza drug (Tamiflu), making star anise a good remedy for cough and flu. Typically, star anise is brewed into a tea and taken after a meal to aid in digestion and relieve bloating or constipation. Its high volatile oil content can be used to alleviate cramps and nausea.

CAUTION: Star anise is used traditionally for colic in infants; however, one must be sure to obtain true Chinese star anise and not Japanese star anise (*Illicium anisatum*), which has been related to cases of toxicity in infants.

---

### ⇥ *Five Spice Powder* ⇤

Star anise is the star of five spice powder mix, which is a foundation for many Asian cuisines. It represents the five elements of Chinese Medicine reflecting the taste quality of sweet, sour, salty, bitter, and spicy.

**MAKES ABOUT ¾ CUP**

1 ounce star anise

1 ounce cloves

1 ounce fennel seed

1 ounce Szechuan peppercorns or
   black peppercorns

1 ounce ground cinnamon

Put all of the spices in a dry iron pan and roast them lightly over low heat for 1 to 2 minutes. Grind the roasted seeds into a powder and store them in an amber glass jar. Use lightly as a rub on chicken or pork or as a variation on pumpkin pie spice blend.

---

## TAMARIND (*Tamarindus indica*)

The pod-like fruit of the tamarind tree is rich in vitamin C, malic acid, tartaric acid, and potassium bitartrate, which gives it tart, laxative qualities making it effective for removing waste from the gallbladder and for treating UTI infections. The pulp is used in Indian cuisine as a sauce or for chutney, and in Mexican cooking it is made into a refreshing iced *agua de tamarindo* (recipe follows). The benefits of consuming the plant include lower cholesterol and blood sugar, healthy skin, decreased appetite, and improved digestion. It is also used along with honey to reduce fevers and soothe sore throats.

### ⇉ *Agua de Tamarindo* ←

**MAKES 8 CUPS**

Tamarind paste is readily available, but if you are lucky enough to collect the pods, begin by peeling the vein off the back and taking the delicate husk off the sticky fruit pod. Plan on using either 4 ounces of paste or about 15 pods. In the meantime, boil 2 quarts of water.

Once you have the paste or the pods ready, place them in a large steel bowl and pour about 1 quart of the boiled water over them, cover, and let sit till it's cool enough to handle. Then with very clean, just-washed hands, squeeze the seeds out of the pods (and any leftover seeds out of the paste) and then strain the seeds and pod waste out to retain the pure thinned pulp. Add the rest of the hot water to taste and sweeten with a little honey or stevia. Cool and drink with ice cubes in the summer or as a hot beverage in the winter. It's very tart but it's the tannins that make it medicinal, so don't sweeten it too much. It also makes wonderful ice cubes and popsicles for children of all ages.

---

## THYME (*Thymus vulgaris*)

The flower, leaves, and oil from the thyme plant are all helpful in treating respiratory infections, bronchitis, sore throat, fever, and cough. A tea made from thyme leaves can be used to reduce the symptoms of a cold. Thyme also acts as a digestive tonic, carminative, and diuretic. Externally, it can be used to soothe inflammation, and oil of thyme applied to the scalp has traditionally been used to encourage hair growth. Thyme contains thymol, a powerful antiseptic that is often added to mouthwash, hand sanitizers, and acne medicine.

### VANILLA (*Vanilla*; *Vanilla planifolia*; *Vanilla pompona*)

Native to Central and South America, vanilla was cultivated by the Olmecs, Totonacs, the Aztecs, and later the Europeans once they colonized the Americas.

Vanilla most commonly refers to the extracted solution made from the seedpods of the orchid genus *Vanilla,* but primarily the *Vanilla planifolia* species. Vanillin is the main flavoring component of the extract, though there are hundreds of other known compounds that contribute to the complex flavor of vanilla. Vanilla is the second most expensive spice in the world after saffron. First fermented and cured for 6 months, the extract is then prepared in a solution of ethanol and water. The extract is used primarily for flavoring pastries and desserts. There is a lot of adulterated and synthetic vanilla extract on the market, so purchasing vanilla pods and making your own extract is the most reliable option for culinary and medicinal use. Vanilla essential oil is used for its relaxing and comforting aromas and is known to enhance libido and cognitive function.

## CONCLUSION

Spices tickle our tongue, grab our breath, sting our fingers, and make our food come alive as they bring us pleasure and reveal hidden stories from the world's cultures. As you explore these recipes, throw yourself into the unknown, pick a sensory response that you seek or a medicine you need, and take a long afternoon to immerse your hands in a mixing bowl of powdered gems and crooked roots that promise to delight, as they bring you health and well-being.

## ⇉ 6 ⇇

# SPIRIT PLANTS

## FINDING THE GODDESS WITHIN

Women the world over have been exploring inner realms for millennia and altering their states of consciousness since our four-footed animal friends first snuffled their way into a mound of fungi and shared their bright-eyed discoveries with us. We have ingested these "spirit plants" to enhance our consciousness, settle our nerves, increase our energy for the fight, and as a route to communion with the divine. Some even suggest that in the Garden of Eden, Eve ate not the apple, but instead the sacred hallucinogen mushroom fly amanita (*Amanita muscaria*), which led her (and Adam) to experience the goddess within, giving rise to what we now call religion.

Spirit plants enter our lives for many reasons and serve many purposes, either planned or discovered. Historically, we have used them with other plants—usually in the context of formalized ritual traditions. These traditions are rooted in women's healing and spiritual practices: the peyote ceremonies among the Wixárikas of central Mexico, the ayahuasca (*Banisteriopsis caapi*) ceremonies from western Brazil, and even the enemas performed using pulque, the fermented substance of the agave plant associated with Mayahuel, the goddess of fertility. We have learned much about spirit plant use from indigenous women across many cultures, and today these plant guides are available to all of us for learning, growth, and celebrating community.

In our ever-changing contemporary lives, we engage in cultural and spiritual practices with plant allies by microdosing mushrooms to aid productivity and mood states, traveling to Amazonian lands for ayahuasca ceremonies, or attending ibogaine clinics offshore to treat opiate addiction—all in order to find meaning and improve our well-being.

These spirit plants, also called "entheogens" (goddess within), enable our inner vision, help us sleep, heal our wounds, and help us transform our deep anxiety about the unknown of impending death by showing us something greater than ourselves.

## SPIRIT PLANT SAFETY

There are many safety concerns we must consider when using spirit plants. In recent years some of these plants have been outlawed or live in the *bardo* of legality— an ever-changing nowhere land of vague laws, where some states or countries allow their use or allow it only under some conditions. Medical or recreational cannabis is perhaps the most important example, but even the plants that make the ayahuasca brew are generally not regulated, yet the main psychoactive component, N,N-Dimethyltryptamine, is classified as a "schedule 1" illegal drug. We also need to be concerned about the adulteration of spirit plants. For example, consider kratom (*Mitragyna speciosa*), which due to growing commercialization has been found commonly to be "cut" with a variety of dangerous drugs, which in some cases has led to death.

When using some spirit plants, especially those that induce hallucinogenic experiences, it is wise to seek out an experienced guide. When using plant substances for mental health recovery, for depression or addiction or trauma, seek out experienced and licensed health providers. Many clinicians, including psychiatrists, are using plant healers in their practice, and their professional support and safe surroundings are likely to ensure positive experiences.

Finally, safety extends beyond the actual spirit plant quality to practicing safety during participation in spirit plant ceremonies. Women can be vulnerable to sexual predators, whether retreat leaders or coparticipants during and after these ceremonies. Advanced planning, research, and specific self-care strategies are essential to ensure safety.

In this chapter I include spirit plants that may be used to lift our spirits (kava, St. John's wort, valerian, and passionflower), as well as plants that cause our spirits to soar, such as entheogens or psychedelics. We use spirit plants for four broad though intersecting purposes: recreation, ritual, therapy, and microdosing. The following list of spirit plants is not exhaustive but more reflective of commonly used or easily accessed plants in the Western Hemisphere. I have not included plants where the safety profile is questionable, or where the plant species itself is endangered and thus should be left alone. As with all plant use, but especially with plants that alter consciousness, I believe that one should carry out inner exploration in the context of ritual with support and a thorough investigation of potential side effects and contraindications unique to each person.

CAUTION: None of these plants should be used during pregnancy or lactation.

### AYAHUASCA, CAAPI, YAGE VINE (*Banisteriopsis caapi*)

The word *ayahuasca* means "vine of the souls" and refers to both the beverage and the vine itself. Ayahuasca is also known as yage, hoasca, or caapi in different cultures. It is a beverage made of the *Banisteriopsis caapi* vine and other psychotropic plants such as chacruna (*Psychotria viridis*), amyruca (*Psychotria carthagenensis*), or chaliponga (*Diplopterys cabrerana*), and it is rich in the spirit molecule dimethyltryptamine (DMT), which is found in hundreds of plants that mimic the neurotransmitter serotonin in the brain. DMT also occurs in the human pineal gland, leading researchers to theorize that DMT is the chemical facilitator of near-death and mystical experiences. All countries have made DMT in its purified form illegal.

Ayahuasca has been used for centuries by indigenous peoples of the Upper Amazon for spiritual and medicinal purposes. Its use spread to Peru where it is used as a medicine for healing. Ayahuasca is often combined with shamanic healing and psychotherapy to recover from drug addiction. Studies suggest no negative effects from long-term usage of ayahuasca. Ayahuasca's legal status in the United States is changing and uncertain.

### CANNABIS (*Cannabis sativa*)

Cannabis is also known as marijuana, pot, herb, mota, and ganga. It is called the "divine nectar" and has been used for treating pain and sleep disorders since ancient times. There are three species of the *Cannabis* plant: *Cannabis sativa*, *Cannabis indica*, and *Cannabis ruderalis*. Tetrahydrocannabinol, or more commonly THC, is the principal psychoactive compound found in cannabis, and cannabidiol, or CBD, is the other major nonpsychoactive chemical, which often balances out THC-induced anxiety.

The women of Thebes, who were twelfth-century silk weavers, used cannabis to decrease sadness and worship the ancient goddess Asherah by burning it as an incense and by anointing the body with cannabis resins. Seshat, the Egyptian goddess of wisdom and writing, is depicted in the temple of Luxor wearing a cannabis-leaf headdress. The Ebers Papyrus marks the use of cannabis for its gynecological benefits, and today CBD-rich vaginal suppositories are sold to decrease the pain of menstruation. Cannabis is beneficial for a variety of issues, including post-traumatic stress disorder (PTSD), depression, anxiety, migraines, and pain. Cannabis targets the memory receptors in the brain, which is probably why people with traumatic memories use it to forget. In the late 1800s, marijuana was used during childbirth for its remarkable ability to cause uterine contractions during labor. Later in the mid-1900s it was used for menstrual cramps and migraine pain. The neurologist Ethan Russo has coined the term "endocannabinoid deficiency syndrome," which he suggests accounts for a variety of symptoms, including PTSD, fibromyalgia, migraines, irritable bowel syndrome, and various eating disorders, all of which can be treated with cannabis.

Cannabis is available in a variety of products with varying amounts of THC and CBD and can be used to smoke and in extracts, edibles, and oils for topical or internal use. As in all herbal medicine and spirit plants, control over the effects is paramount and always begins with a low dose. The method of delivery should also be considered. For example, one may have less control over the effects of eating and digesting cannabis than those of other methods such as tincture or smoke, which can be regulated more effectively. There is some evidence that CBD-rich cannabis can be used to treat severe neurological illnesses and act as an anticonvulsant in epilepsy. Given the varieties of epilepsy and challenges involved with standard treatment interventions, using cannabis for epilepsy warrants collaboration with a neurologist. Finally, considerable literature suggests delaying use of cannabis (unless indicated for medical purposes) by adolescents until neurological development is complete in early adulthood.

### ↠ Bhang Lassi with CBD Oil ↞

Bhang lassi is a traditional beverage that is made by grinding cannabis flowers into a paste and mixing the paste with milk, honey, and spices. This lassi uses CBD oil (not THC) to ease the pain of menstrual cramps, manage chronic pain, or induce sleep. Test out the effects of the lassi before you need it and when you are not required at work or an event. Consider a dose range of 2.5 to 20 milligrams for chronic pain and a range of 40 to 160 milligrams for sleep disorders. I always suggest starting out at 5 milligrams of CBD oil and slowly increasing it until an effect is felt. Digesting cannabis with food takes longer than other forms of consumption, but its effects last longer as well.

MAKES 1 SERVING

½ cup whole milk yogurt

½ cup coconut milk

2 tablespoons almond butter

¼ cup raw local honey

1 thumb fresh ginger or ¼ teaspoon
    ground ginger

1 pinch garam masala

1 teaspoon rose water

5 milligrams edible CBD oil

Add all the ingredients to a blender and blend until combined. Add ice if desired.

---

## CHOCOLATE (*Theobroma cacao*)

Chocolate, called the food of the gods, is medicine, mood booster, and the elixir of love. It is one of the great gifts Mexico has given the world. Chocolate (without sugar of course) is rich in antioxidants and minerals for heart and brain health. It can be added to food to enhance flavor or taken on its own. It makes a good substitute for an afternoon coffee as it provides energy without overstimulating.

**CAUTION:** Due to its high arginine levels, chocolate should be taken only on special occasions and in very small quantities by people with gastroesophageal reflex disease (GERD) or those who develop herpes simplex outbreaks. In these cases, in advance of eating chocolate, take a dose of up to 3 grams a day of lysine to counteract the effects of arginine.

## COFFEE (*Coffea arabica*)

Coffee is a drug, not a beverage, so use it like one! Drinking coffee in small doses is a mild antidepressant that enhances mood and aids focus, attention, and productivity. In larger amounts it can contribute to anxiety and heart palpitations. Women metabolize coffee more slowly than men, which is often why we need to drink it earlier in the day. Seven ounces of brewed coffee contains about 80 to 135 milligrams of caffeine. Caffeine binds to adenosine receptors in the brain, which, without the presence of caffeine, usually cause drowsiness and depression in the central nervous system. In the presence of caffeine, upon binding to these sites, nerve cell activity speeds up, creating a stimulating effect. Consuming coffee is associated with lower risk of heart disease, certain cancers, diabetes, liver disease, and cognitive disorders like Parkinson's. Coffee can be ingested via the oral or rectal route. When used for enemas it aids liver detoxification (see page 43). Only organic coffee should be consumed to avoid chemicals used in growing and processing beans.

### IBOGA (*Tabernanthe iboga*)

Native to Central Africa, the *Tabernanthe iboga* plant is a rainforest shrub that is endangered from overharvesting. The indigenous peoples of Gabon, who are adherents to the Bwiti religion, chew the bark in initiation rites and for healing. The psychoactive alkaloid ibogaine, found in the roots of the plant, eliminates symptoms of withdrawal and reduces cravings for opiates. Individuals with opiate addictions often experience a release from dependence shortly after ingestion. There are many clinics located around the world that offer treatment with this spirit plant.

CAUTION: Ibogaine is classified as a controlled substance by many Western nations, and it is not approved for addiction treatment in the United States. Use of iboga must be done with an experienced guide as it can lead to powerful and sometimes dangerous reactions.

### KAVA KAVA (*Piper methysticum*)

Kava kava, or simply kava as it is more often called, is effective as an anti-anxiety herb and can be used instead of benzodiazepines. A South Pacific island plant and member of the pepper family, kava is both medicinal and sacred. The name *kava*, or *awa*, means "bitter." Kava contains chemicals called kavalactones, or kavapyrones, which are responsible for most of kava's pharmacological effects, including increased gamma-aminobutyric acid (GABA) transmission, central nervous system depression, and norepinephrine pooling. Kava also reduces fear and anxiety, making it useful for PTSD. It is also a muscle relaxant, and it enhances cognitive performance and reduces menopausal anxiety.

Kava is available in an alcohol-based extract or in capsules. Doses range from 100 to 400 milligrams (60 percent kavalactone per capsule), 3 times daily. Most people can start with one 200 milligram capsule (60 percent kavalactone) and increase it to 2 if necessary, up to 3 times a day. People who are sensitive may prefer using an extract in order to measure by drops and achieve more specifically the minimum dose required for effect.

While some individuals use kava for sleep, the stimulating effects of kava suggest that it is best used for anxiety during the day. When experiencing anxiety and insomnia, use kava during the day, and the "three sisters of sleep"—hops, valerian, and passionflower—at night.

Kava has been used in rituals for millennia with no apparent adverse reactions. The aqueous extract of kava was found to be safe, with no serious adverse effects and no clinical hepatotoxicity.

CAUTION: Case reports of liver damage and death associated with kava use led to warnings about the use of kava. However, the World Health Organization issued a report that clinical trials and experimental studies reveal no hepatic toxicity from kava and the case reports of illness suggested evidence that adulterants or contaminants were the likely culprit. After exhaustive studies, the warnings on kava were removed by many countries. As with all herbal medication, it should be used at therapeutic doses. Kava is contraindicated in people taking benzodiazepines or antipsychotic drugs and in patients with Parkinson's disease. Kava should be discontinued at least twenty-four hours before surgery because of its possible interaction with anesthetics.

### KRATOM (*Mitragyna speciosa*)

Native to Southeast Asia, kratom is a traditional medicine that is a stimulant at lower doses and an analgesic at higher doses. It is used to decrease pain and anxiety, improve mood, and increase stamina. Its primary use has been as an aid to opiate withdrawal. Unlike opiates it does not appear to depress respiratory function.

CAUTION: Significant concerns exist with kratom use due to adulteration, as manufacturers may cut their product with other herbs or potent synthetic opioid drugs, hydrocodone, and morphine.

### MORNING GLORY (*Ipomoea tricolor*; *Ipomoea violacea*; *Rivea corymbosa*)

When I lived in the jungle, I was greeted each morning by a large ranging vine with beautiful round flowers that spread across my front window. By midday the honeybees were collecting their nectar. The plant is native to Mexico where *Rivea corymbosa* is called ololiuqui, meaning "round things," in reference to the seeds. The morning glory seeds contain a mild hallucinogen used in traditional practices among many indigenous peoples in Mexico. The vine itself is called "green snake," ostensibly because of its endless growth and twining. Traditionally, the seeds are used in the context of shamanic facilitation to explore questions or concerns.

### PASSIONFLOWER (*Passiflora*; *Passiflora edulis*; *Passiflora incarnata*)

Passionflower is a tropical vine plant native to Central and South America. A gentle and effective nervine and sedative, *Passiflora incarnata* contains chrysin, an anxiolytic that rivals the effects of benzodiazepines and is safe to use to treat stress and anxiety in children. Passionflower also reduces asthma symptoms and arthritic pain and stiffness. The leaves are used as a sedative and for menstrual distress, and some species have entheogenic seeds. Use as a tea or capsule 200 to 400 milligrams as a nervine and up to 600 milligrams for sleep.

### PEYOTE (*Lophophora williamsii*)

Peyote is a cactus that grows in the deserts of Central Mexico and as far north as Texas. It is called the Divine Herb and Medicine of God. The peyote origin story is that of the wounded healer. In it, a woman is lost and starving and needs help for herself and her people. She finds peyote, ingests it, and is healed and able to find her way. She then takes peyote back to her people.

The Wixárikas use peyote in salves to treat pain and scorpion stings and to receive messages from the gods. Peyote is also used traditionally in Mexico to reduce fevers and to promote lactation. The bitter-tasting fresh or dried peyote "buttons" are made into a tea, chewed, or eaten in powdered form.

The Native American Church is an officially recognized religion in which the peyote cactus is used as a sacramental medicine. Participation in the ceremony is often used to support sobriety and requires abstinence from alcohol and drugs. Peyote is a vulnerable medicine plant on the International Union for Conservation of Nature Red List of Threatened Species.

### SALVIA (*Salvia divinorum*)

Salvia is member of the mint family and native to Mexico. Also called the Shepherdess, the leaves of salvia are smoked, chewed, or brewed and lead to intense short-lived trance responses such as alterations in visual perception and conception of space and time. Salvia is rare in the wild and is now cultivated around the world.

This spirit plant is used in low doses to treat headaches and pain and for treatment-resistant depression to improve mood and increase self-awareness. Salvia ritual ceremonies focus on protection, meditation, and divination. The primary active component in salvia is salvinorin A, which is readily absorbed via the mucous membranes of the mouth and is considered one of the most potent naturally occurring hallucinogens. Smoking the leaves is the most effective mode of use. Start with a very a low dose, ⅛ to ¼ gram, to see how you respond. Many people react poorly to salvia (it affects opiate receptors in the brain), so it is important to educate yourself prior to use and to ensure that you are in a very safe place with a nonusing guide present. Salvia is legal in most of the United States.

### ST. JOHN'S WORT (*Hypericum perforatum*)

St. John's wort is used for depression, anxiety, and obsessive-compulsive disorder. It has consistently been found to be as effective as selective serotonin reuptake inhibitor (SSRI) medications in the treatment of mild to moderate depression. Most studies have explored a dose of 900 to 1,500 milligrams a day in 3 divided doses via capsule or tincture.

CAUTION: St. John's wort can produce mania and photosensitivity in humans. Avoid exposure to strong sunlight when you are taking it. Do not use with pharmaceutical antidepressants. St. John's wort can be used to withdraw from SSRIs under the guidance of a professional.

## TOBACCO (*Nicotiana tabacum*)

*Nicotiana tobacum* is a member of the *Solanaceae* (nightshade) family and used traditionally by indigenous peoples in rituals to communicate with the gods and as an antidote for poisons and animal bites. Tobacco was used as an entheogen and ritual plant by American Indians at the time of contact with Europeans. Back in the 1700s, smoke from tobacco was used as an enema to revive drowning victims who were presumed dead; hence the saying, "Don't blow smoke up my butt!"

Nicotine is a highly addictive stimulant that releases dopamine, the pleasure chemical, in the brain and enhances mood and cognitive function. The use of tobacco as an addictive substance rather than a sacred plant is emblematic of many plant medicines when used outside of ritual, spiritual context.

Recent research has identified some benefits of nicotine for people with Alzheimer's. There is a growing movement to restore use of sacred tobacco among native peoples as a method of relinquishing addictive tobacco use.

### ⇉ *Protocol to Withdraw and Cease Nicotine Use* ←

Herbal medicines are integral to tobacco addiction cessation programs. Here is a list of herbal methods that can help in the process of giving up tobacco.

- Make or obtain a tincture of lobelia, licorice root, oat milk seed, St. John's wort, and passionflower (see Herb Pharm in the "Resources" section). Take 40 drops 3 times a day.

- Obtain licorice root sticks and suck on them instead of a cigarette when you want to place something in the mouth. CAUTION: Licorice can raise blood pressure, so monitor your blood pressure.

- Every 3 to 4 hours, eat foods that stimulate dopamine like chocolate, coffee, bananas, walnuts, and high-protein and healthy-fat foods rich in choline such as eggs, liver, and fish.

- Apply lavender-infused coconut oil to the skin and dry brush skin 3 times a day.

- Use black pepper essential oil in a diffuser.
- Receive the National Acupuncture Detoxification Association, or NADA, protocol.
- Do aerobic interval training for 5 to 10 minutes whenever needed throughout the day. Deep, heavy breathing reduces cravings.

---

### VALERIAN (*Valeriana officinalis*)

Cats love the nasty smell of valerian, which is why it is called *hierba de los gatos* ("the cats' herb") in Mexico. Valerian incense has long been used to protect against evil spirits. It is most valuable to aid sleep disorders, reduce anxiety, and relax tense muscles. Because valerenic acid binds to the GABA receptors, valerian is used in place of benzodiazepines in addiction treatment. Historically, the root of valerian was used as an aphrodisiac.

CAUTION: Do not take valerian while using alcohol or benzodiazepines.

## CONCLUSION

Women have always been the holders of sacred space, sharing brews and mixtures for communal rituals and individual passage into realms of healing. According to the ancient story of the maiden goddess of vegetation, Persephone was "abducted" into the underworld (inner world) as a result of eating the entheogenic narcissus flowers. In the 1950s, the Mazatec *curandera* (healer) Maria Sabina introduced to researchers outside of her village the sacred *Psilocybe mexicana* mushroom that the Nahua call *teonanacatl*, or Flesh of the Gods. She said, "There is a world beyond ours that is far away, nearby, and invisible. And that is where God lives, where the dead live, the spirits and the saints, a world where everything has already happened and everything is known." But Maria Sabina also came to regret her inclusion of foreigners into her ceremonies since they brought with them the psychedelic revolution that destroyed the way of life in her village and the meaning of "little saint children," as she called the mushrooms. This is but one example of the complexities involved in accessing and using spirit plants and the need to understand our responsibility as wise women and imparters of sacred knowledge. As we seek personal growth and healing we may ask, "How does our quest affect not only us, but others, nature, and the environment?"

⇹ **7** ⇷

# HERBAL MEDICINES FOR LIFE'S CYCLES, HEALTH, AND DIS-EASE

n this chapter I explain herbal medicine use for many of the biological processes we experience during our life cycle and for specific physical and mental dis-eases we may experience. Notice that I have hyphenated the word *dis-ease* in this chapter to call attention to its root meaning: being "out of ease." Herbal medicines help bring us back into ease and contribute a broad range of remedies as they help us maintain balance and heal illness. Where indicated I also include complementary interventions such as nutrition, movement, massage, and hydrotherapies that enhance treatment efficacy and improve our quality of life.

## TRAUMA, HEALTH, AND HERBAL MEDICINE

It is not possible to talk about our health as women without considering trauma and adverse childhood experiences. Traumatic experiences occur commonly in the lives of women and children. Such experiences change our physical, emotional, and spiritual health, often for life. As a traumatologist, I treat the effects of trauma on women's physical and mental health. I have spent my career working with women suffering from chronic health problems that most often had their beginnings in the experience of childhood trauma. While not every illness is a result of trauma (for example, a head cold or stubbed toe), the effects of trauma and stress on all aspects of personal functioning cannot be denied. Every body organ dysfunction and many illnesses can be traced to the disruption of psychological, endocrine, immunological, digestive, and musculoskeletal systems caused by trauma. Exposure to traumatic events during childhood can be recognized in adults as a very high risk factor associated with eating disorders, fibromyalgia, autoimmune disorders, digestive upset, pain, depression, insomnia, chronic fatigue, substance abuse, cardiovascular disease, and disruptions along the reproductive life cycle. Herbal medicine, as I explain, has much to offer us in our recovery from trauma.

## HOW TO USE HERBAL MEDICINES
## FOR HEALTH AND ILLNESS

When using herbs and botanicals for physical or mental health, remember to choose several herbs that complement and synergize each other instead of taking a high dose of just one herb. Start slowly, using one herb at a time so you can tell the specific effects and then add in the other herbs, unless you are already starting with a predefined compound. In the following sections I give you options for several herbs along with some foods, nutrients, and other healing methods. It is helpful to rotate the herbs that you take. For example, take an herb for 3 weeks or 3 months and then try another adaptogen or analgesic. Not every herb will be right for your body, so if you don't feel results, or a particular herb makes you feel badly, try a different herb or an herbal compound. It doesn't mean the herb doesn't work at all; it just may not be right for you.

Finally, as a licensed psychotherapist, massage therapist, and herbalist I believe in the power of telling our stories as a path to healing. Just as psychotherapy alone has its limitations, so too does looking to herbs for all of our healing. However, just telling our story with words may not be enough. We may need to give our body the chance to tell its story. It is also important to remember that our needs change throughout our lives and working with professional guides and experienced herbalists can help us navigate those changes and enhance our health along the way.

# DIGESTION

Digestion involves many stages. Once we smell, chew, and swallow our food and herbs, they travel a complicated route through our body. The esophagus delivers partially broken-down food to the stomach and from there the liver and pancreas kick in, and the food passes into the gastrointestinal tract, or "second brain," which makes use of our nutrients and generates mood chemicals. Finally the peristaltic action of the digestive track—our rhythmic push—moves digested food into the colon for further absorption of vitamins, and then waste is available to be passed out the rectum. Along the way, any nook and cranny of the intestines can cause concern: a stitch or fiery pain, bad bacteria, or a bubble all can cause distress.

Digestion normally occurs without a hitch when the nervous system is relaxed. Herbal medicine works best when we take some time to rest and relax and allow our digestive juices to flow. One of the first steps for preventing digestive problems is to make sure our liver is functioning well and that we help it when it weakens.

## SOAPING UP THE LIVER AND GALLBLADDER

The gallbladder is a small sac connected to the liver that stores bile. When digestion needs support the gallbladder releases the dark green to yellowish-brown fluid into the small intestine where it helps to emulsify fats. Bile is like soap. Think of trying to wash your pan without soap after you stir-fry with coconut oil. The coconut oil simply stays in the pan. Soap breaks oils and fats down so water can serve as a solvent. This is the function of bile. It breaks down fats and makes them available for nutritional use by the body and brain.

Nature in her wisdom has given us many herbs to support bile function, so essential is it to brain, body, and mental health. Mixing bitter greens like dandelions, arugula, and epazote is an ideal way to break down fats while you eat. Sometimes despite our best efforts we end up with sludge or even crystalized stones in the gallbladder, which inhibit the emulsifying effects, and we experience nausea. Many of our healing plants contain saponins, soap-like substances that help to emulsify fats, so it is best to include these plants in our diet.

The gallbladder can also fill up with crystals and stones as a response to pregnancy, hormone replacement, increased estrogen levels, or just too many trans fats (unsaturated fatty acids). However, surgically removing the gallbladder is like throwing out the garbage pail, instead of cleaning it. Avoid gallbladder surgery at all costs. Cleaning out the gallbladder "pail" can be accomplished with good-quality oils, in particular a regular dose of virgin cold-pressed olive oil mixed with lemon juice, garlic, and ginger. The "Spring Cleanse" I suggest on pages 41–45 is designed to keep this waste moving. I do this cleanse at the change of every season. Add orange and lemon zest to your salads, make your own digestive "bitters" like dandelion and arugula, and don't be afraid of fats; if you cut down too much, the gallbladder takes a nap and won't push out any waste for you.

## ⇻ *Lecithin Liver Smoothie* ⇺

This liver/gallbladder recipe supports a happy liver and gallbladder. This recipe combines a decoction for liver health that you may drink alone or add to the smoothie. The lecithin in the smoothie has the added benefit of helping to remove fat from the liver in cases of nonalcoholic fatty liver disease and the green tea and berries are antioxidants.

MAKES 1 GALLON, ABOUT 16 SERVINGS

**FOR THE DECOCTION**

1½ ounces dandelion leaf and root
1½ ounces Oregon grape root
1½ ounces milk thistle seed
1½ ounces schisandra berry
1 gallon water

**FOR THE SMOOTHIE**

4 ounces coconut milk
1 tablespoon non-GMO sunflower lecithin granules or powder
½ teaspoon green tea powder
1 cup frozen berries of your choice

In a large stock pot, add the dandelion leaf and root, Oregon grape root, milk thistle seed, and schisandra berry to the water and decoct (see page 19). This decoction will make enough for about 16 servings, and last for about 2 weeks of daily use. Store the decoction in the refrigerator.

To make a daily smoothie, add 1 cup of the decoction to the coconut milk, green tea powder, sunflower lecithin granules, and frozen berries to a blender and blend until combined. Drink 1 serving a day for 30 days. Do this cleanse every 3 months, or 4 times a year.

As an alternative preparation to the decoction, you can add 10 drops from each of these herbal extracts into your daily smoothie.

# STRESS: I JUST CAN'T STOMACH IT!

Stress contributes to all kinds of digestive upset, including problems with stomach acid, heartburn, gastroesophageal reflux disorder (GERD), nausea, inflammatory bowel disease, colitis, diarrhea, and constipation. All of our herbal remedies for these dis-eases will be enhanced with stress reduction. Because stress also contributes to inflammation (which can easily lead to depression and anxiety), reducing stress will help any herbal medicine we use do its job even more effectively. Let's consider how herbs can help each of these imbalances.

## STOMACH ACID AND GERD

GERD occurs when stomach contents rise into the esophagus. Stomach acid problems and GERD frequently, though not always, go together. More often, the problem begins with gastritis, and over time GERD evolves from chronic gastritis. Conventional medicine suggests that too much stomach acid causes problems, so it needs to be suppressed. However, natural medicine asserts that GERD is really a problem of too *little* stomach acid available to adequately digest protein, coupled with eating too many refined carbohydrates and acidic foods that exacerbate the symptoms. One of the best herbal remedies to naturally increase hydrochloric acid in the stomach is gentian tea.

Interestingly, people with post-traumatic stress disorder (PTSD) have higher rates of GERD and chronic pain. The use of aspirin or nonsteroidal anti-inflammatory drugs (NSAIDs), can also damage the stomach lining, encouraging us to look for a healthy approach in herbal painkillers and anti-inflammatories, which I consider later in this chapter.

## TREATING HEARTBURN, NAUSEA, GERD, AND HIATAL HERNIA

Nausea has two main causes (besides morning sickness): heartburn coming from the stomach and dysfunction of the liver/bile. If the nausea is coming from the liver, you can use ginger and peppermint tea for relief. However, these herbs might worsen stomach acid and GERD, in which case chamomile and licorice root are soothing alternatives.

GERD can be a symptom of hiatal hernia, and a hiatal hernia can be a response to chronic GERD. To treat a hiatal hernia, apply an ice pack to the stomach just below the breastbone for 15 minutes before a meal. Dietary changes are also necessary and herbs promise results. Note that the usual acid blockers like proton pump inhibitors should be eliminated, as stomach acid is necessary to metabolize nutrients and medicinal metabolites from foods and herbs. There is also evidence that acid blockers increase the risk of dementia.

There are two main steps to address this complex of imbalances: soothe the inflamed tissue and then slowly support enough stomach acid to digest efficiently. First eliminate all acidic foods from your diet, especially coffee, tea, citrus, and tomatoes, along with all flour, wheat, and sugar. Then undertake a 45-day process of using the two most important herbs for reducing and eliminating symptoms of GERD: licorice root and a combination of cabbage juice extract and chlorophyll. To make the cabbage mixture, juice ¼ of a green cabbage (vitamin U) along with a little dark lettuce and take a shot glass of it 3 times a day. If you do not have a juicer, you can purchase a pill of dehydrated cabbage juice and chlorophyll. Since GERD also results from stress, chamomile and nervine herbs will help you relax. You may also benefit from elevating your upper body after you eat. Remember to not eat for at least 2 hours before bed.

After the 45-day treatment, your stomach and esophageal lining will be much improved, and you can begin to supplement with 15 drops of gentian tincture with each meal. However, do not return to the acid foods just yet; you may actually need to consider them as treats rather than daily foods. If you require coffee, make cold brewed coffee, since it produces less acid, and never drink it on an empty stomach.

## THE SECOND BRAIN

A healthy gut is essential to overall physical and mental well-being and herbal medicines are ideal to restore the gut. Your intestinal tract is called the "second brain." This is due in part because your intestines direct so many actions of the body and work in cooperation with the first brain in your head. Intestines actually make even more chemicals for the brain than the brain makes for itself. Think about your gut as your inner garden. When it is out of balance, not much will grow, but when it is healthy and you give it plenty of plant fibers (soil) and fermented foods (nutrients), its teeming, healthy bacteria digest food efficiently and nutrients are absorbed through intestinal walls into the bloodstream, which generates an abundant supply of neurotransmitters (bright flowers) to support our mood and relaxation.

### INTESTINAL PERMEABILITY
Stress, NSAID use, alcohol, and unrecognized gluten and casein sensitivity can all inflame the sensitive mucosa of the small and large intestines, which is often the

start of dis-ease contributing to obesity, liver issues, allergic reactions, pain, type 2 diabetes, and autoimmune disorders. Healing the second brain supports all your efforts toward good health. Think of the difference between a new sponge and one that has been used to clean dishes for six months. It's a rough idea of the difference between a healthy mucosal barrier and one that is frayed and can't do its job.

### ⇉  *Music to My Mucosa Smoothie*  ⇇

Your intestinal mucosa will love this smoothie as it soothes inflammation and provides healing nutrients. Each of these ingredients supports the healing process. The green tea and curcumin in the turmeric are powerful anti-inflammatories, which are potentiated by the black pepper. Ginkgo has been shown to heal intestinal mucosal cells, and the glutamine is an important fuel for intestinal lining.

CAUTION: Ginkgo biloba extract can increase the efficacy of warfarin, so consistent use of ginkgo should be done with professional advice and monitoring warfarin levels. However, ginkgo does not appear to effect any other medication interactions. This recipe contains a low dose of turmeric, which should not interefer with warfarin or other blood thinners. The maximum dose of turmeric a day is considered 2,000 milligrams. However, it is always wise to seek medical advice when mixing herbal medicines with pharmaceuticals.

**MAKES 1 SERVING**

½ cup hemp or almond milk

½ cup strong green tea

1 cup raspberries or blackberries
   (fresh or frozen)

40 milligrams ginkgo biloba extract
   (with 24 percent ginkgo flavonoid
   glycosides)

5 grams glutamine powder

1 teaspoon fresh turmeric juice or
   1 tablespoon ground turmeric

Dash of freshly ground black pepper

½ teaspoon black currant seed oil or
   evening primrose oil

Add all the ingredients to a blender and blend until combined. Drink daily for 1 month.

## INFLAMMATORY BOWEL DISEASE

Colitis and Crohn's disease are inflammatory processes that can be helped with dietary and herbal interventions. Getting tested for food allergies and sensitivities, including celiac disease and gluten sensitivity, is important. Many people who are sensitive to gluten are also sensitive to dairy products. Fermented food is a superb remedy for healing the gut as are simple vegetable broths rich in minerals and bone broths full of soothing collagen and glycine. Eating mono meals (meals made up of just one food, such as a raw fruit or vegetable) can help to ease digestion.

To heal the colon, rotate the following herbal remedies, using one or two each day so you use each remedy a few times throughout the week. Pay attention to how each remedy makes you feel in order to fine-tune your protocol.

- Drink 1 cup of Slippery Elm Bark Tea (page 97). You may also add a sprinkle of powdered cinnamon.

- Drink 1 cup of Golden Milk (page 100) made with a nut or seed milk.

- Drink 1 cup of chamomile fennel tea. To make: add 1 heaping tablespoon of fresh or dried chamomile flowers and 1 teaspoon of fennel seed and simmer gently in 1½ cups of boiling water for 15 minutes. Strain and drink.

- Drink the It Takes Guts Smoothie (recipe follows).

## → *It Takes Guts Smoothie* ←

Collagen protein powder is an easily digested protein that is derived from marine sources or beef and provides soothing support and nutrition for a sensitive gut. This smoothie could be one of your meals each day.

**MAKES 1 SERVING**

1 cup strong chamomile tea or almond milk (without carrageenan)

2 tablespoons collagen protein powder

½ frozen banana

½ teaspoon powdered probiotics

½ teaspoon ground turmeric

½ teaspoon boswellia extract

½ teaspoon evening primrose oil

10 drops stevia (or to taste)

Add all the ingredients to a blender and blend until combined. Drink daily as a nourishing, easily digested meal.

## CONSTIPATION

Constipation is a digestive symptom where fecal waste is hard and difficult to pass through the colon and eliminate. There are several factors that may contribute to constipation. Anything that affects peristalsis, the rhythm of the colon, can cause constipation: lack of exercise and stress, lack of fiber in the diet, and slower transit time through the colon, which can also happen with age.

General ways to ease constipation begin with drinking plenty of water. You can also add a tablespoon of chia seeds or psyllium husk to a daily glass of water. Also try adding more fiber to your diet, including fruits, vegetables and their skins, and grains like oatmeal. Oral magnesium (400 milligrams a day) or vitamin C (up to 2,000 milligrams a day) are mild laxatives that can help.

### → *Prune Tea* ←

Prunes are a delicious and often underrated dried fruit that are a perfect remedy for constipation. Prunes are rich in phenols that are natural laxatives. Fill a glass pint jar halfway with prunes and then pour 1½ to 2 cups of hot Earl Grey tea over the prunes, filling the jar to the top. Sprinkle some orange zest on top and let cool uncovered. Store in the fridge for up to a week and eat a few of the prunes and some of the Earl Grey syrup each morning with breakfast. For severe cases of acute constipation, make a tea of senna leaf or cascara sagrada.

## DIARRHEA

For diarrhea due to stress, irritation, or a stomach virus use slippery elm bark tea. Slippery elm bark is safe for children and is soothing and nourishing. Sipping on some tea with a little added cinnamon will soothe the mucous membranes and slow peristalsis. Eating a little banana or rice with cinnamon and a few raisins or sipping a simple chicken broth for a day or so will also help. When diarrhea is due to food poisoning take ¼ cup of liquid bentonite to absorb the toxic bacteria, followed by very strong chamomile tea to soothe the inflammation.

## HEMORRHOIDS

Swollen and inflamed veins in the rectum or anus can occur because of constipation or frequently during pregnancy and can be painful and/or itchy. The following recipe is the perfect antidote and should be used at the first hint of a hemorrhoid.

---

⇸ *Banana Peel for Hemorrhoids* ⇷

The peel from a banana is rich in antioxidant and anti-inflammatory quercetin and vitamin C. Remove the peel from the banana and lay it face up, so the white pulp is showing. Place a piece of waxed or parchment paper on a tray next to the peel. Use a spoon to scrape the pulp off the peel and form the pulp into small oval shapes that can easily be inserted into the anus. Make a few dozen ovals and place them on the tray with the waxed paper; then place the tray in the freezer. When frozen, each oval can be placed gently into a small container and kept in the freezer. Insert 1 to 2 ovals into the anus at night (wear a protective pad if needed). Do this treatment for a minimum of 3 nights.

---

# HYPOGLYCEMIA AND TYPE 2 DIABETES

When I first arrived in Mexico I noticed that cinnamon (canela) tea was the breakfast beverage of choice and was also drunk before bedtime. However, over time this tradition gave way to drinking milk, coffee, and even a soft drink like a cola instead. Since cinnamon is an effective herb for keeping diabetes at bay, I wondered whether losing the ritual of drinking cinnamon tea every morning heralded the onset of the diabetes epidemic in Mexico, which has some of the highest rates of diabetes in the world and continues to worsen with "modernization." Traditional herbal practices teach us a great deal about health: A cup of cinnamon tea is a healthy way to start the day and a soothing way to end the evening. Cinnamon contains methylhydroxy-chalcone, a polyphenol compound that improves insulin sensitivity.

The way we manage glucose in our blood affects nearly every aspect of our health. Consuming too much sugar in the form of refined sugars, carbohydrates, and alcohol leads to three stages of imbalance and then illness. The first stage is hypoglycemia. Hypoglycemia occurs when sugar intake triggers the repeated and excessive release of insulin. In these cases blood sugar rises fast and high and then drops sharply and can cause dizziness, trembling, fatigue, irritability, and confusion. This is followed by insulin resistance, type 2 diabetes, and can eventually lead to type 3 diabetes, the new term for Alzheimer's disease. In hypoglycemia and insulin resistance, the body cells begin to ignore the message that insulin sends out, which is, "Let glucose in." It takes a larger and larger amount of insulin to get the cells to respond to this direction, and when the cells do not respond, glucose stays outside of the cells, in the blood. When the level of glucose in the blood continues to rise, this becomes hyperglycemia, high blood sugar, or type 2 diabetes. Too much blood glucose is also inflammatory, and even if we do not develop diabetes, it contributes to metabolic syndrome and can become a major factor in physical pain, cardiovascular disease, and poor mental health.

There are many herbs that can prevent or treat this cascade of events. Our goal is to reduce or eliminate refined sugar intake, slow the uptake of glucose once we eat (think fiber), help our cells use their glucose effectively (yes, the brain needs glucose), dampen systemic inflammation, and support the health of our liver and nervous and vascular systems.

Finally, stress is a major factor in glucose metabolism, so the adaptogenic herbs that reduce stress and enable the adrenal glands to function better will be part of the repertoire. Eating a diet of protein, good-quality fats, and small amounts of complex carbs every 3 hours helps stabilize the ups and downs of hypoglycemia. Most people with glucose problems benefit from eliminating most (or all) grains from their diet, or if necessary eating them only on rare occasions. Herbs and spices for hypoglycemia and diabetes can help stabilize blood sugar by supporting the pancreas, liver, and adrenal glands.

## HERBS FOR TYPE 2 DIABETES AND HYPOGLYCEMIA

Herbs used to treat type 2 diabetes should actively enhance circulation and eye health, and in later stages, reduce edema, enhance kidney function, support cognitive health, and provide neuropathic pain relief. Herbs used for hypoglycemia and diabetes may reduce the levels of medication required, so monitoring dosage is advised. There are many fine pharmaceutical-grade herbal-vitamin compounds on the market to complement your home herbal remedies. Look for a compound that also combines the minerals chromium and vanadium.

## BLOOD GLUCOSE REGULATION

American ginseng is a blood sugar regulator that boosts energy levels and increases the stimulation of the pituitary gland, which releases hormones that regulate blood sugar. Add 15 to 20 drops of ginseng tincture to liquids, or take 400 milligrams, 3 times a day after meals. Mugwort stimulates the pancreas to create more insulin. Add 5 drops of tincture to liquids, 3 times a day. Bitter melon lowers blood glucose and can be juiced, eaten as raw fruit, or used as an extract.

## FOR THE LIVER

Dandelion root and milk thistle improve liver and pancreas function. Drink a decoction half an hour before meals or keep some in the fridge and add it to your smoothies daily.

The gymnemic acid in gymnema leaves suppresses cravings for sugar and balances blood sugar levels. Gymnema capsules should have at least 25 percent gymnemic acid. Take 5 to 10 minutes before a meal 3 times a day every day, to stablize blood glucose levels.

## ANTIOXIDANTS

One of the effects of hyperglycemia is that high blood glucose is toxic to the vascular system and leads to oxidative stress, which is like rust on a car. These reactive oxygen chemicals are also called free radicals and they damage our cells, leading to systemic illness. They are a major factor in the aging process. Daily supplies of antioxidants from foods and herbs are protective because they scavenge these free radicals and neutralize them.

Green tea is a powerful antioxidant that can be used daily to slow glucose uptake. Fibers from vegetables and low glycemic fruits like apples, cherries, and pears, along with ground seeds like flax and chia, slow glucose uptake and should be part of every meal. Ground flaxseeds also lower blood sugar and blood pressure. Fenugreek seeds are high in soluble fiber, and a tea from the seeds is hypoglycemic and slows digestion and absorption of carbohydrates. Curry leaves (*Murraya koenigii*) support normal levels of glucose and enhance liver enzymes. The bitter leaves of neem, or margosa (*Azadirachta indica*), enhance insulin receptor sensitivity and lower blood glucose levels. The tender shoots of neem leaves can be juiced or chewed raw, or 1 to 2 teaspoons of dried neem leaf powder can be added to your daily smoothie.

# STRESS, DEPRESSION, INSOMNIA, AND FATIGUE

While stress, depression, insomnia, and fatigue are often treated separately, they frequently co-occur and effective treatment will work on all four symptoms. Chronic or acute stress usually precedes the development of depression and/or anxiety. Traumatic stress events can lead to complex trauma, PTSD, and chronic anxiety symptoms. Women who did not sleep in safe homes as children or do not do so as adults frequently have trouble relaxing into deep sleep at night, always ever vigilant. Indeed, the latest research suggests that African American women actually get less restful sleep and have higher rates of high blood pressure than white women, and this is believed to be due to the stress of being always on guard in a society that does not ensure their safety. Understanding social causes of stress can inform our use of herbal medicines with family, friends, and neighbors and reinforce our commitment to actively engaging in social justice for all our sisters.

## STRESS

Stress may originate from the home or from society in general. Many women and children, whether living in rural or urban regions, are under the stress of domestic violence. Women of color, lesbians, and bisexual and questioning women, as well as transgender and gender nonconforming individuals, are subjected to daily stress at home, at school, at work, and in health care.

Acute stress is not generally a health concern; our body and mind respond to the stressor by mobilizing energy to help us cope in the short term. However, when stress becomes chronic, it disrupts our biological rhythms, depletes our energy, and makes us vulnerable to illness. Stress is inevitable in our lives and during these periods, if we nourish the body with good-quality foods, enriching minerals, and adaptogenic herbs and support our capacity to cope by resting, then we can often weather the stress storms that life brings with minimal negative effects on our health.

Adverse childhood events like physical, emotional, or sexual abuse or growing up around caregivers with addictions can cause chronic stress and require that we engage in daily acts of self-care that nourish our brain, mind, and body. We know that many physical health problems are related to these early life stressors: autoimmune illnesses, fibromyalgia, chronic pain, insomnia, digestive upset, depression, and addiction. Knowing these causal roots reduces our shame and illuminates a path we may forge, using herbs and foods as our ally medicines, to brave the route of the wounded healer.

## HEALING STRESS WITH ADAPTOGENS

Adaptogens help us to adapt to stress by restoring the biological capacity to cope and respond. They are also called "metabolic regulators" because they help us to adapt to environmental stressors. The herbal treatment to restore balance for all of these related symptoms is very similar, and we need only ask ourselves, "Do I need a bit more of an herbal anxiolytic or sedative, or an herbal antidepressant?"

# INSOMNIA AND SLEEP DISORDERS

Sleep is the foundation for all mental health; a disrupted circadian rhythm underlies depression, PTSD, bipolar disorder, PMS, bulimia, and insomnia. Hence restoring the capacity to sleep deeply is the first step to take in treating these disorders. Begin with restoring the natural biological cycle, the circadian rhythm, and move your "clock" closer to going to bed no later than 11:00 PM and waking up no later than 7:00 AM. Licorice root tea (1 cup a day) and vitamin B-12 (methylcobalamin) help to regulate our 24-hour clock.

## INSOMNIA

There are two major types of insomnia: one is where you can't fall asleep, and the other is where you fall asleep but awaken several hours later and have trouble falling back to sleep. Using nervines and sedatives can help the first type. Addressing hypoglycemia, which can be significant cause of awakening, can treat the second type. To stabilize glucose metabolism throughout sleep, eat a small snack of fat, protein, and carbohydrates just before bed. Bioidentical oral progesterone (not topical) is a good natural sedative that helps you get to sleep and stay asleep once perimenopause begins. In addition, the use of melatonin can help reset circadian rhythm (it does not aid sleep per se). Each night before 11:00 PM, spray up to 3 milligrams of liposomal melatonin under the tongue.

## THE THREE SISTERS OF SLEEP AND KAVA

Hops, valerian, and passionflower, which I call the "three sisters of sleep," help with both types of insomnia. They are frequently combined for their synergistic effect for the treatment of sleep disorders. However, they may not reduce very high levels of anxiety or acute panic. In these cases, turn to kava. It comes as an alcoholic extract or in capsules. Start with the extract so you can easily measure a small dose and observe your response. If using capsules (containing 75 milligrams of kavalactones), start with 1 and increase to 2 as necessary.

CAUTION: The use of hops should be monitored for its estrogenic effects in hormone dependent cancers. Note that kava can be stimulating and keeps some people awake.

### FIBROMYALGIA

Fibromyalgia is more common in women than men. It is a musculoskeletal and sleep disorder characterized by general pain with fatigue, sleep, memory, and mood problems. Fibromyalgia often emerges after periods of intense psychological stress, PTSD, physical trauma, surgery, or infection. I have worked with women with fibromyalgia in my clinical practice for over forty years, and I have observed that it always occurs when there has been a history of adverse childhood events and complex trauma. Treatment benefits can be achieved from herbs such as the cannabinoids (topical and internal), anti-inflammatories, and rubefacients like capsaicin, along with the generous use of healthy fats, detoxification strategies, gentle massage, and aromatherapies. Treatment takes time and patience and must be multifocal, supporting the psyche, the immunological, endocrine, and musculoskeletal systems, and circadian rhythm.

## DEPRESSION

Depression is another way to describe learned helplessness. Action helps to overcome the sense of learned helplessness, whether it is making an herbal bath or an extract for a friend or some sachets for elders or our children. Using herbal medicine not only heals the body and mind; it heals the political alma (the soul). Self-care is the soul of social justice. Our self-care is a political act that then spreads to helping others. It is part of claiming and identifying who we are and what we need for ourselves and our families.

Depression is not about a deficiency in serotonin; it is about inflammation. Depression and pain often co-occur, and this is because being in pain is depressing, and because inflammation underlies both symptoms. Alongside the numerous herbs and spices to use daily for inflammation and depression is the lesser-known herb tarragon, which contains rubidium, a trace element that lifts mood, so use it generously in your salad dressings and seasonings. Rubidium is also found in coffee, but it is only beneficial when taken as a coffee enema. It is also well established that 1 hour of aerobic exercise is very effective for depression and will complement the following protocol.

During depression it is difficult to mobilize self-care, so begin slowly and simply, ask for help, and keep your protocols and meals simple. Use slow cookers and smoothies to get the greatest benefit from the least amount of effort, and focus on self-care as a ritual. Check your vitamin D levels, as low vitamin D can cause or exacerbate depression and pain. Coffee or rhodiola can be used as a short-term booster, but the underlying imbalances should be addressed as well. If you are a vegetarian, you may benefit from more acidifying foods that include vinegars and vinegar baths. Each day add 2 tablespoons of apple cider vinegar to your salads and 1 cup of vinegar to a whole body (or foot) bath and soak for 20 minutes.

Make or purchase an extract with the following combination of antidepressant herbs and mood stabilizers. They combine support for the nervous system and enhance parasympathetic dominance and adrenal function. Take for up to 3 months.

### ANTIDEPRESSANT HERBS

- St. John's wort
- Passionflower
- Saffron
- Schisandra

- Gotu kola
- Rosemary
- Korean ginseng
- Milky oat seed

## FATIGUE

There are many connections between stress, depression, chronic fatigue syndrome, adrenal fatigue, and fibromyalgia. Adaptogens, nervines, anti-inflammatories, and topical rubefacients will help all these symptoms.

Adrenal fatigue usually arises after a period of prolonged stress. The release of adrenal hormones follows circadian rhythm and when our lifestyle upsets this rhythm (like working the night shift), it leads, over time, to fatigue. The adrenal glands sit atop each kidney in the middle/lower back area. They are responsible for the hormone production that plays a role in sexual health, our 24-hour sleep/wake cycle, blood pressure, inflammation, and fluid and mineral excretion. To support the adrenal glands, use sea salt and warming spices like cayenne, cinnamon, cardamom, and cloves in your diet.

### CHRONIC FATIGUE SYNDROME

Chronic fatigue syndrome, also called systemic exertion intolerance disease and myalgic encephalomyelitis, is a condition characterized by extreme tiredness and exhaustion without any diagnosed, underlying cause. It is more common in women, and sleep or rest does not help. Chronic fatigue may be triggered by chronic stress, a viral infection, or environmental exposures. Antiviral herbs like licorice along with coenzyme Q10 and a Myer's cocktail IV can be added to the adaptogenic protocol to support immune function. Herbal powders that target retroviruses include skullcap, bitter melon, reishi, green tea, nettles, and olive leaf.

# IMMUNE SYSTEM HEALTH

The immune system is central to our health as women, and immunomodulatory fungi such as turkey tail bring it into balance. The thymus gland that lies just beneath the upper part of the breastbone in the middle of the chest is a major organ that acts as a teacher, training white blood cells how to do their job. Over time and as we age, the thymus gland "retires." The Greek word *thymos* refers to "spiritedness." The immune system is very responsive to stress—it can be hyperactive, a bit paranoid, and overreactive, which can lead to allergies and autoimmune disease, or it can be underactive and sluggish, which leaves us vulnerable to viral and bacterial infections. Acute stress causes our immune system to prepare to attack any perceived enemies, but over the long term, stress can either keep our system activated, which leads to autoimmune illness, or simply exhaust it.

Here, I examine some of the more important health concerns we have as women relating to immune function along with suggestions for treatment.

## HERPES SIMPLEX VIRUS

Herpes simplex is a contagious virus passed from person to person by direct contact. There are two types: oral herpes (HSV-1) and genital herpes (HSV-2), both of which cause uncomfortable blisters on the surface of the skin. After the initial infection, the herpes virus stays in the system, and a flare-up will reoccur in the event of stress, decreased immune function, or sunlight exposure. In more serious, rare cases, the herpes virus can affect the brain, nervous system, and eyes. Intensive use of antiviral herbs is the foundation for treatment. Reducing triggers such as chocolate, wheat, and almonds can help, along with lysine supplementation. Intravenous vitamin C and short-term, high-dose vitamin A can suppress the virus.

## HPV AND CERVICAL DYSPLASIA

The treatment of human papillomavirus, or HPV, and cervical dysplasia are fraught with controversy. HPV refers to hundreds of types of sexually transmitted skin-to-skin contact viruses that pose a health risk. Nearly 80 million people in the United States have some form of the virus, but most do not experience any symptoms, and women experience symptoms more than men. For most people the virus poses no problems. In a small percentage of people, it can lead to genital warts or to cervical cancer, which can be terminal. It is not always obvious that a sexual partner has the virus.

Effective treatment should combine professional treatment and self-care at home. Like many health care options there are pros and cons to each, and elements that may factor into your individual situation include time, resources, and health beliefs.

Regular Papanicolaou tests, or Pap smears, can identify any cervical cell changes and lead to a program to enhance immune function. Many women who wish to bear children want alternatives that reduce risk of conventional treatments, yet herbal and natural medicines also pose some risks.

Self-care methods at home that use herbal medicines and foods should complement care and oversight provided by a professional where cervical dysplasia is present due to HPV. Traditional Chinese Medicine can identify and treat systemic imbalances, including the use of specific herbs to support your ability to suppress and counteract the effects of a virus. The foundation of any treatment of cancerous cells or prevention of abnormal cell progression to cancer can include the use of high-dose oral pancreatic enzymes, preferably as part of a protocol under the care of a professional.

## TOPICAL OINTMENTS AND SUPPOSITORIES FOR HPV

Green tea extracts applied topically in ointments limit the progression of HPV as well as cervical dysplasia, and green tea suppositories can also be helpful. A probiotics-rich diet with garlic and onions enhances the function of the immune system.

## LIVER SUPPORT AND VIRUS SUPPRESSION

Indian gooseberry fruit (*Phyllanthus emblica*) is a valuable Ayurvedic fruit and herb that can be eaten pickled, fresh, or dried and is available in capsule form. It may be used daily for liver and immune support, and it has shown inhibitory activity against HPV. Licorice root also supports immune health and targets HPV.

## FOODS THAT SUPPRESS HPV

Eating raw or slightly cooked foods from the *Brassica* genus (broccoli, cabbage, bok choy, brussels sprouts, and cauliflower) may suppress the HPV virus. Indole-3-carbinol is one of the metabolites formed during the breakdown of glucobrassicin, a compound found in cruciferous vegetables that is associated with anticancer activity. Indole-3-carbinol supplements have been explored in the treatment of cervical/vulvar cancers and recurrent respiratory papillomatosis. Because the effects are strongest in raw brassicas, most daily servings should be raw and consumed along with a small amount of lightly cooked vegetables daily.

## ESCHAROTIC TREATMENT OR LOOP ELECTRICAL EXCISION PROCEDURE FOR HPV AND CERVICAL CANCER PREVENTION

Escharotic treatment refers to applying an herbal escharotic agent to the cervical lesion topically that burns the lesion and destroys cancerous or precancerous cells. Proteolytic enzymes and a variety of herbs are applied directly to the lesions. This treatment is often done instead of the loop electrical excision procedure, which has potential complications as well as benefits. There is a significant debate about the utility and dangers of escharotic treatment, and some herbalists and naturopath advocates are vehemently opposed to it. Like most medical choices where risk is involved, the decision becomes a matter of personal philosophy. Finances may affect options and since there are risks inherent in both methods, the risk/benefits should be addressed with health care providers. Trusting an intervention is often linked to trust in the provider and feeling heard and understood by her. There is no easy answer to choices for treatment but obtaining several expert opinions can help you decide your next steps.

## SHINGLES AND POSTHERPETIC NEURALGIA

Shingles (herpes zoster) is a reactivation of the varicella zoster virus (the virus that also causes chicken pox), most commonly seen in older adults or people with poor immune function, though occasionally in children.

Postherpetic neuralgia is the most common symptom of shingles and frequently causes severe nerve pain. I have treated many people in my clinical practice with postherpetic neuralgia, and herbal treatments can serve as an important part of a repertoire of medicine for reducing nerve pain. For some people the pain is considerable, and herbs will play an adjunctive role to medicines like gabapentin by allowing a reduction in medication dose.

Four types of herbal actions help in the management and recovery of shingles and include topical and internal applications: anti-inflammatory, immunomodulatory, adaptogenic, and analgesic. Topical applications include licorice root gel (have your compounding pharmacist make it for you), which can be applied to shingles lesions as an anti-inflammatory, and capsaicin cream, which can also be purchased over-the-counter as Zostrix neuropathy cream (0.25 percent capsaicin) or, if a stronger dose is required, it can be compounded by prescription up to 2 percent at a compounding pharmacy.

Cannabis strains that are rich in varying ratios of THC, CBD, and terpenoids provide options for anti-inflammatory and analgesic topical application of gels or creams to herpetic lesions and for use orally as oils and tinctures for neuropathic pain. Consult with your local cannabis pharmacy about these special strains and options. Ginseng and schisandra act as adaptogens and modulate immune function, and fungi like reishi and shiitake are immunomodulators that can be incorporated into daily diet or taken with other fungi like agarikon (*Laricifomes officinalis* and *Fomitopsis officinalis*), which Paul Stamets of Fungi Perfecti suggests as an antiviral available as a concentrated powder in capsules. Some experimental work has also been done using apitherapy (bee venom injections used to reduce pain). This procedure requires a licensed clinician experienced in and knowledgeable about this protocol.

The shingles vaccine can provide protection against the disease, and although shingles can still occur in spite of vaccination, it does so with fewer symptoms and for a shorter duration.

## ACUPUNCTURE AND HERBAL TREATMENTS FOR IMMUNE HEALTH

There are two types of treatments for immune support: herbs that provide gentle daily support and powerful immune boosters and virus suppressors that can be used just before or during flare-ups. The following sections provide treatment suggestions for both types along with an exercise to wake up your immune system.

**IMMUNE HEALTH HERBS FOR DAILY USE**

Use a single herb or a combination of the following herbs in capsule or extract (garlic may be used fresh and elderberry may be used in a syrup) to enhance your daily immune health:

- Echinacea
- Reishi
- Schisandra
- Garlic
- Astragalus
- Elderberry

**IMMUNE HEALTH HERBS FOR ACUTE ILLNESS**

When you're under immune stress, you can take extracts for short periods of time (2 to 3 weeks) that include the following herbs:

- Echinacea root
- Licorice root
- Osha root
- Goldenseal

### → *Immune Boost Soup* ←

This soup provides an effective and delicious food for immune support that you may create in your healing kitchen.

**SERVES 4 TO 6**

- 1 cup shiitake mushrooms (fresh or dried)
- 1 cup maitake mushrooms (fresh or dried)
- 6 cups vegetable, chicken, or bone broth
- ½ cup burdock root
- ½ onion, chopped
- ¼ cup astragalus root (dried or fresh)
- 1 thumb fresh ginger
- 1 thumb fresh turmeric
- 3 cloves garlic

1 small piece kombu

1 cup finely chopped Napa cabbage

Freshly ground black pepper

Pinch of ground cayenne pepper

If the mushrooms are dried, rehydrate them. To a large stockpot, add the broth and bring to a simmer. Add all the ingredients except for the Napa cabbage and the black and cayenne peppers. Bring to a boil and then turn it down and gently cook for 60 minutes on very low heat. If using a slow cooker, simply cook the soup on low for 8 hours. Divide the cabbage between each serving bowl and pour the soup over. Sprinkle cayenne pepper and black pepper on top to taste. If using only vegetable stock (no fat) add a touch of sesame oil (*Sesamum indicum*) at the finish to enhance absorption of the nutrients.

---

### → *Exercise: Jane Beats Her Chest* ←

The acupuncture points of the immune system are centered above the thymus gland, which is in middle of the chest, and about 1 inch down from the juncture of your collar bone where there is a soft spot. A simple tapping on these points sends a message that says, "Wake up! I am feeding you healing herbs and foods to bring balance. Please do your job!" Tap these points for about 60 to 90 seconds while breathing in and out repeating, "Ha, ha, ha, ha" over and over as you tap. This is also called the "Jane beats her chest" point (Jane, as in Tarzan's companion).

---

# AUTOIMMUNE ILLNESSES

Autoimmune disease is an umbrella term for a range of diseases in which the body's immune system mistakenly attacks its own healthy cells. The most common autoimmune syndromes are rheumatoid arthritis (RA), lupus, Sjögren's syndrome, Hashimoto's thyroiditis, celiac, multiple sclerosis, and type 1 diabetes.

Women have significantly higher rates of autoimmune diseases. There is a relationship between exposure to stress and trauma early in life and the development of autoimmune disorders, suggesting that reducing stress and addressing the multifaceted effects of trauma can "reverse engineer" the hyperreactivity of the immune system. There is also evidence that inflammatory food, like sugar and flour and chemical and pesticide exposure make one more vulnerable to these diseases.

Herbs can help suppress and manage symptoms of these autoimmune diseases, decrease or eliminate medication, improve the quality of life, and serve as an important part of the overall plan for recovery. The foundation for the treatment involves the use of immunomodulatory and anti-inflammatory herbs and essential fatty acids from plants and fish that help to keep the whole system lubricated.

Immunomodulators are herbs like licorice and echinacea that either selectively enhance or suppress the immune system. Dietary fats like omega-3 fatty acids (flax, hemp, and fish oils) and gamma linolenic fatty acids such evening primrose oil, black currant oil, borage oil, and black cumin seed oil are all powerful anti-inflammatories, immunomodulators, and emollients that synergize the benefits of herbs.

## SJÖGREN'S SYNDROME

In Sjögren's syndrome, the immune system attacks the salivary and tear glands causing them to stop producing sufficient moisture. Sjögren's commonly co- occurs with RA, lupus, or celiac disease. Nine out of ten people with Sjögren's are women. Herbs for Sjögren's syndrome should include immunomodulators and potent emollients.

Sea buckthorn seed and its fruit (*Elaeagnus rhamnoides*) are strong emollients and anti-inflammatories rich in phytosterols, carotenoids, omega-7, and vitamin E. The oil from the buckthorn seed can be applied topically or be taken internally by adding it to smoothies and salad dressings or as soft gel oil extracts (2,000 milligrams a day).

→ *Treating Dry Mouth and Dry Eyes* ←

Oil pulling using coconut or sesame oil can help dry mouth, and it's easy to make an herbal emollient to treat dry eyes. You can make a strong tea to use as eyedrops by combining equal parts of eyebright and chamomile. Be sure to strain the tea in a very fine strainer and then bottle it in a sterilized glass jar and refrigerate. The strong tea will last in the fridge for up to 5 days. To use, pour the tea onto a clean cotton ball or use a dropper and drop a few drops into each eye.

The application of bioidentical testosterone cream around the eyelids near the tear ducts is also useful for stimulating the tear ducts.

## LUPUS

Lupus affects many body organs and can include symptoms of skin rashes, joint and muscle pain, fatigue, malaise, anemia, mood disorders, and inflammation of the cardiovascular and respiratory systems. In severe cases, lupus can lead to renal failure, neurological disorders, miscarriage, cardiovascular disease, and death. Because the symptoms of lupus mirror many other diseases, it is often misdiagnosed. It is common for people with lupus to have periods of acute illness (flare-ups) followed by periods of remission.

Herbs used for lupus include nettles and gotu kola. Thunder duke vine (*Tripterygium wilfordii*), often referred to as thunder god vine, has also been used successfully with lupus to reduce swelling and pain. However, it does have some side effects when used longterm so be sure to rotate it with different plants.

CAUTION: Alfalfa should be avoided by people with lupus since it can overstimulate the immune system.

## RHEUMATOID ARTHRITIS

RA is an inflammatory, autoimmune disease that attacks the lining of joints and in some severe cases, the lining of other body systems, including the cardiovascular and respiratory systems. Women are three times more likely to have RA than men. The most common symptoms of RA are pain and swelling around joints, which over time can lead to bone erosion and joint deformities.

Plant essential fatty acids from evening primrose (1,000 milligrams a day) and borage oil (1,000 milligrams a day) are the foundation of treatment along with elimination of gluten and casein. There is one theory that RA can arise from chronic infection and treatment employs the use of antitbiotics successfully. As an alternative to pharmaceutical antibiotics, take one 50 milligram capsule of the plant "antibiotic" emulsified oil of oregano before bed for 30 days and repeat every 3 months. The oil is a potent antibacterial and anti-inflammatory, so do not use beyond 30 days at a time. Following internal use, a few drops may be added to a carrier oil and rubbed on inflamed joints. Make sure you supplement with probiotic-rich food, following internal use of oregano.

## THYROID HEALTH

When problems arise with the thyroid, it is usually due to underactivity, or hypothyroidism, but it can also be caused by overactivity, or hyperthyroidism. Hypothyroidism occurs when the thyroid does not produce enough hormones, which leads to weight gain, depression, constipation, hair loss, and dry skin. Hyperthyroidism occurs when the thyroid produces too much of the thyroid hormones, causing insomnia, anxiety, weight loss, and heart palpitations.

Hashimoto's thyroiditis is an autoimmune disease that causes hypothyroidism. The disease is much more prevalent among women than men and can remain asymptomatic for a long period of time. The disease, often occurring in response to gluten sensitivity, causes antibodies generated in the immune system to attack the thyroid gland, slowly damaging the thyroid. Symptoms of the disease include fatigue, weight gain, joint and muscle pain, and depression.

Unhealthy diet, chronic stress, environmental toxins, and infections can all contribute to thyroid imbalance. Conventional treatment usually includes thyroid hormones (porcine or synthetic) and autoimmune dietary and herbal medicines. Iodine is also essential for thyroid health and eating iodine-rich plants like seaweeds and adaptogenic herbal teas complement the use of porcine thyroid treatments.

&#8658;  *Adaptogenic Extract for Hypoactive Thyroid*  &#8656;

Add 15 drops each of ashwagandha, gotu kola, eleuthero, and milk thistle extracts to a little water and take twice a day. Assess thyroid response after use for 3 to 6 months.

## HERBS AND MEDICINAL FUNGI FOR AUTOIMMUNE HEALTH IN THE GUT

Like all chronic illness, autoimmune diseases benefit from healing the "second brain," the microbiome (natural microorganisms) of the gut. Burdock root and dandelion root are beneficial as both contain inulin, a prebiotic fiber that helps to feed and proliferate healthy gut bacteria, which in turn stimulate the healing of the digestive tissue. Calendula, a vulnerary, heals damaged tissue throughout the digestive tract while also reducing inflammation. Medicinal fungi such as cloud mushroom (turkey tail), cordyceps, and reishi are effective immunomodulators and can be included in the diet as a fresh source or as capsules.

## HERBS FOR INTERNAL USE TO DECREASE PAIN
## AND INFLAMMATION IN AUTOIMMUNE DISORDERS

Test the effects of these herbs one at a time or in combinations to assess your individual response.

**Birch bark** (*Betula lenta*): A tea made from this bark is rich in betulinic acid, which has a powerful anti-inflammatory activity.

**Cat's claw bark** (*Uncaria tomentosa*): Use a tea, tincture, or capsule as an immunomodulator and anti-inflammatory. Eat with food as stomach acid releases tannins in the bark.

**Andrographis** (*Andrographis paniculata*): Use an extract or capsules. This herb has an anti-inflammatory effect and improves RA-related anemia. It is called the "King of Bitters" because every part of the plant is extremely bitter tasting, which suggests why it is effective as an antifungal and antibacterial and in treating digestive problems.

**Sarsaparilla root** (*Smilax ornata*): This herb is an anti-inflammatory that can be taken as a decoction, extract, or capsule.

**Boswellia:** Use in capsule form for pain and inflammation.

**Dong quai:** Take a tincture of the dried root for muscle and joint pain.

**Feverfew:** Use a tincture, tea, or capsule to decrease inflammation and pain.

**Ginger tea:** Use fresh or dried as a juice or tea as an anti-inflammatory and digestive stimulant.

**White peony root** (*Paeonia lactiflora*): Peony is an immunomodulator and anti-inflammatory. Use a tea, tincture, or capsule.

**White willow bark:** This bark is rich in salicin, which is a natural analgesic and reduces inflammation. Use as a powder or in capsules. **Caution:** People with asthma may be intolerant of salicylate rich herbs and foods.

## → *Autoimmune Beverage* ←

**MAKES 1 TO 2 SERVINGS**

In a small saucepan, add 1 teaspoon each of celery seed, devil's claw root, birch bark, and dandelion root to 4 cups of boiling water. Gently simmer for 15 minutes and then strain. Drink daily to reduce connective tissue inflammation.

## → *Golden Paste* ←

Turmeric can be used for joint health. You can take it in capsule form of 400 to 600 milligrams 3 times a day, but remember that to be effectively absorbed, turmeric requires black pepper and a little fat, so include those in your diet as well.

This paste, great for curries, salads, steamed vegetables, and smoothies that call for turmeric, can also be applied topically to swollen joints for a minimum of an hour or even overnight during sleep. It stains, so the best way to handle it is to apply it to the affected joint and then cover it with two layers of light cotton flannel. When you're done, save the flannel in a plastic bag in the fridge until you want to use it again. To remove the stain from your skin (or you can live with it during your treatment period), mix equal parts baking soda and lemon and gently scrub.

**MAKES 1 CUP**

½ cup ground turmeric
1 cup water
1½ teaspoons freshly ground
   black pepper

6 tablespoons virgin cold-pressed olive
   or coconut oil

To a small saucepan, add the turmeric and water. Heat on low, simmering for 20 minutes until it turns into a paste, and then mix in the pepper and olive oil. Add the paste to a small jar and refrigerate it for daily use for up to a month.

# TOPICAL HERBAL RECIPES TO DECREASE PAIN AND INFLAMMATION IN AUTOIMMUNE DISORDERS

## ↠ *Arnica Compress* ↞

Prepare a decoction of arnica root. Dip a soft cotton cloth in the liquid and apply it to the affected area for 30 to 45 minutes to reduce swelling and pain.

## ↠ *Ginger Cayenne Conifer Massage Oil* ↞

This oil is beneficial for musculoskeletal, neuropathic, or burning pain.

**MAKES 1 CUP**

½ cup virgin cold-pressed olive oil

½ cup hemp seed oil

Large handful of freshly picked
　　conifer needles

1 tablespoon ground cayenne pepper

1 tablespoon ground ginger

To a saucepan, add the olive oil, hemp seed oil, and conifer needles and simmer gently for 2 hours on very low heat. After simmering, strain well through a cheesecloth. If you don't have access to the needles, you can add pine needle extract once the oil cools.

Pour the oil in an amber glass jar, add the cayenne pepper and ginger, and screw the lid on tightly, letting it sit in a sunny warm window for 2 weeks. Strain well and then bottle. Rub on painful limbs, joints, and muscles as needed. (If you do not have the time to wait 2 weeks then you can return the conifer needle infused oil to the heat and gently simmer the powdered herbs for 2 hours on the lowest possible heat, then strain and bottle.

As another option you may have a compounding pharmacist mix a topical capsaicin cream at a stronger dose or with a mild anesthetic to achieve a dose level that is right for you.

# HEADACHE

There are many types of headaches, including tension, migraine, cluster, and hypnic headaches. Headaches can be caused by numerous underlying issues including muscle tension, food allergies, serotonin imbalance, and dehydration. Here I provide some general approaches to use with all types of headaches along with interventions for specific causes.

## ⟫ *Dehydration* ⟪

Dehydration is a common factor in all types of headaches and increasing water intake is the first step. To calculate how much water you should drink a day in ounces, take your body weight and divide it by 50 percent. So a 200-pound woman requires 75 to 100 ounces a day.

## ⟫ *Mustard Footbath* ⟪

Headaches can result from changes in cerebral blood flow or vessel constriction, and a simple self-care method is to do a mustard foot soak. Add a tablespoon of ground mustard (grinding fresh mustard seed is best, but commercially ground mustard will do in a pinch) to a bucket of hot water that is deep enough to cover up to your ankles. Massage some virgin cold-pressed olive oil into your feet and ankles and then soak them in the mustard water for 30 minutes. The heat from the water and the mustard will draw down the vascular congestion and release constricted blood vessels in the head, bringing blood flow to the feet and alleviating the pain. Do the bath once a day during a headache and a few times a week to help prevent one.

## MIGRAINE HEADACHES

Migraines can be particularly challenging, as they have different and multiple causes. Food sensitivities—particularly to gluten or foods high in salicylates—can be a culprit as can stress, hypoglycemia, or changes in barometric pressure. Many people choose to relocate to regions with less variability in pressure to avoid not only migraines but muscle aches and joint pain. I recommend the use of the mineral lithium orotate. Unlike the dangerous pharmaceutical lithium carbonate, lithium orotate is nature's gift to us. It relieves headaches, gives us the giggles as it boosts our mood, and protects neurons in the brain. Lithium can be dosed from 5 to 25 milligrams a day, or you can go on vacation and soak in lithium-rich mineral springs in New Mexico, Washington State, Texas, or Mexico. Lithium also helps the rare hypnic headaches occurring primarily in older women.

In addition to lithium orotate, use these other effective herbal treatments include the following:

- Combine 25 to 150 milligrams of 5-hydroxytryptophan (5-HTP), the amino acid precursor to serotonin and 50 milligrams vitamin B-6.

- 750 milligrams St. John's wort twice a day.

- 125 milligrams of dried feverfew leaf from authenticated feverfew containing at least 0.2 percent parthenolide, 3 times a day.

- Cannabis (balanced tetrahydrocannabinol [THC] and cannabidiol [CBD]) in both an analgesic and antiemetic form. For migraines you might consider a formula with 50 percent THC and 50 percent CBD. Formulations vary greatly by producer. Consider a formula containing 10 to 35 milligrams cannabidiol per milliliter and use for pain as needed.

- 250 milligrams sangre de grado/dragon's blood (*Croton lechleri*) extract starting at 4 times a day and increasing up to 500 milligrams 4 four times a day.

- Women who develop migraines at perimenopause may benefit from prescribed bioidentical estrogen or estrogen-precursor herbs like hops.

Some self-care measures, like drinking enough water, taking a mustard bath, or using 5-HTP and B-6, or lithium orotate and magnesium, can be used daily for prevention. It is important to try each remedy, one at a time, and give it time to work and see how you respond.

The use of herbs like feverfew, St. John's wort, sangre de grado, and cannabis can be applied upon headache onset. Use an herb for a day or a week or a few months at the onset of the headache in order to test whether it's right for you. If you have other symptoms for which an herb can be helpful, then choose that herb first so that you can minimize the number of herbs you use for your well-being. Make sure you check any contraindications for use of these herbs.

# REPRODUCTIVE AND GENITOURINARY HEALTH THROUGH THE LIFE CYCLE

My earliest studies on the use of herbs in midwifery were conducted in the jungle of Mexico and expanded on later when I was in public health graduate school. These studies included the ways in which women's methods of healing were forced underground in the late nineteenth century in the face of an increasingly male-dominated medical profession that sought to "medicalize" childbirth.

As I attended childbirths in the jungle and studied history, I discovered that one of the most important medicines given to women during childbirth in the early twentieth century was called scopolamine. Given as an amnesic, scopolamine is a tropane alkaloid drug derived from the *Solanaceae* (nightshade) plants such as henbane (*Hyoscyamus niger*) and jimsonweed (*Datura stramonium*). Scopolamine was often mixed with morphine ostensibly to ease the difficulty of childbirth, but it actually induced what was called a "twilight sleep." Rather than experiencing pain relief, women frequently suffered terribly during birth, but then they remembered nothing about the experience. The hallucinatory nature of scopolamine led to confusion and women would thrash about, half conscious, and were often tied to their beds while in labor to mediate the vigorous movement. When I read the medical notes on my own birth, I saw that my mother was given scopolamine along with Demerol during my birth. This "cocktail" was administered to nearly every woman who had a hospital birth in the United States well into the 1960s.

While tracing the origin of scopolamine use, I discovered that the compound is found in plants used by wisewomen to make what was called "flying ointment." These hallucinogenic "flying" plants include deadly nightshade (*Atropa belladonna*), henbane, henbane bell (*Scopolia carniolica*), jimsonweed (*Datura stramonium*), and mandrake (*Mandragora*). Women healers (often called witches or sorceresses) made this ointment in order to "fly and see."

Fortunately, today women are reclaiming the many choices for birthing and for healing. While the use of scopolamine as a hallucinogen is not advised, many women are handcrafting these special ointments for their medicinal and ritual value. While tracing scopolamine use in women's childbirth, I learned two important lessons: Though many of our drugs derive from plants, when only a single component of that plant is extracted and concentrated and used in ways nature did not intend, it can cause dangerous side effects that damage women's lives. I also learned about the persistence and resilience of women's wisdom, and that we carry on the knowledge of our foremothers—we need only look just beneath the surface information about how many drugs are used today to find the seed that holds the power for healing.

# MENSTRUATION

There are a lot of variations in menstrual cycles, and it's important to know your own cycle well. Experiencing cramps, PMS, shorter or longer cycles, or excessive bleeding can all be bothersome; however, these symptoms can often be improved with diet and herbal medicines. Here are rituals, exercises, teas, and fomentations to ease the many forms of menstrual distress.

## AMENORRHEA

Primary amenorrhea is when menses fails to occur by fifteen years of age. Secondary amenorrhea is when menstruation has ceased for at least three months (if your cycle was regular) or six months (if your cycle was irregular). Stress, polycystic ovary syndrome (PCOS), thyroid dysfunction, or low body fat are common causes. The following emmenagogue is an effective treatment.

### ⇒ *Herbal Emmenagogue* ⇐

**MAKES 8 CUPS**

Add 2 teaspoons each of chasteberry, partridgeberry, rue, black cohosh, motherwort, and white peony to 2 quarts of boiling water. Let sit for an hour, strain, and store the tea in the fridge, warming gently before use. Drink 1 cup twice a day for 4 days to bring on menstruation.

## DYSMENORRHEA

Dysmenorrhea is when menstruation is painful. The following protocol combines herbs and nutrients to use throughout the month and specifically during menses.

### ⇒ *Dysmenorrhea Protocol* ⇐

- Take black currant seed oil (2,000 milligrams), magnesium (400 milligrams), and vitamin B-6 (100 milligrams) every day to reduce cramps during menstruation.

- Drink a mixture of fresh ginger, chamomile, cramp bark, and skullcap tea 3 days before your flow begins and continue to drink it during menstruation.
- Add cinnamon to your foods during menstruation.

---

### ⇾ *Topical Treatments for Dysmenorrhea* ←

- Obtain a kansa wand, an Ayurvedic bronze tool designed for self-massage on the face and abdomen. Add 6 drops of rose essential oil to a tablespoon of liquid magnesium lotion. Rub the lotion on your belly and slowly use the kansa wand, moving in small clockwise circles over the area of discomfort.
- Rub some almond oil on your lower abdomen first and then rub a few drops of peppermint essential oil over the almond oil.
- Add 1 cup of magnesium sulfate (Epsom salt) and 8 drops of lavender essential oil to a bath and soak for 30 minutes a day starting 3 days prior to your flow.

---

## PREMENSTRUAL SYNDROME (PMS)

PMS describes a group of physical and psychological symptoms experienced by some women just prior to the onset of menses each month. Aproximately one-third of all women experience some form of PMS, and for many, those symptoms are severe enough to affect the quality of their life. PMS is related to shifts in estrogen and progesterone during the menstrual cycle. Estrogen excess, progesterone deficiency, and low magnesium levels are all contributing factors. Symptoms include bloating, headaches, cramping, fatigue, anxiety, and depression. Keeping a journal to track one's own experience of PMS can be a useful tool to identify patterns in the menstrual cycle and can better target herbal and self-care interventions.

### ⇾ *Treatments for PMS* ←

- Pine bark extract from the French maritime pine tree (*Pinus pinaster*) is sold as Pycnogenol and used for PMS and menstrual pain. Use 40 to 200 milligrams once or twice a day. Start with smaller dose and increase as necessary.
- Begin taking ashwagandha (1 gram, 3 times a day as capsule) and dandelion (4 grams of dried leaf, 3 times a day as an infusion) to support hormonal balance and help to release fluid tension 7 days prior to onset of menses and through completion of the cycle. Fluid retention is exacerbated by dehydration as the body strives to retain water, so hydrate well during menses.

- Add magnesium (up to 400 milligrams a day) and vitamin B-6 (100 milligrams a day) into your monthly routine along with black currant seed oil (1,000 milligrams a day). As you near perimenopause and your cycles shorten, intramuscular injections of magnesium and B-6 provide relief by regulating cycle length.
- Obtain at least 20 minutes of sunlight (or full spectrum light) each day, reducing sunglass use.

## URINARY TRACT INFECTIONS

Urinary tract infections (UTIs) occur when bacteria enter the urethra and multiply in the bladder, causing painful urination, feelings of not entirely emptying the bladder, pelvic pressure, discomfort, and blood in the urine. If UTIs are not treated in a timely manner, the infection may spread to the kidneys, which causes nausea, chills, fever, and back and side pain.

Not all UTIs are the same. "Honeymoon cystitis" is the result of sexual intercourse, and UTIs are commonly experienced by postmenopausal women in response to low levels of estrogen. Estrogen enhances the vaginal wall integrity, which provides a protective barrier against bacteria.

Among older women who are confined to bed or institutionalized, there can be chronic, low-grade, often asymptomatic UTIs, which can affect mental function. These women should always be assessed for UTIs.

Herbal treatment of UTIs can often be successful; however, if pain or fever persist after treating an acute and painful UTI for 24 to 48 hours with herbs, seek medical advice.

### ⇉ *UTI Prevention* ⇇

- Integrate cranberry juice (no sugar added) into your diet at least a few times a week, and add cranberry concentrate to your salad dressings with olive and hemp oil, lemon, and garlic.
- Eat fermented herbs or vegetables rich in probiotic cultures at least 3 times a week.
- Apply bioidentical estrogen cream to the vaginal walls 3 times a week (for postmenopausal women).

## ⇒  *UTI Treatment*  ⬅

- Take 15 drops of each extract of echinacea, uva ursi, buchu, old man's beard (*Usnea*), and corn silk 3 to 4 times a day.
- Mix 2 grams of D-mannose powder into a glass of water twice a day.
- Eat garlic soup and fermented vegetables.

CAUTION: If the infection does not clear up or if you have severe pain or a fever, seek medical attention. Sometimes antibiotics are necessary.

# INTERSTITIAL CYSTITIS/PAINFUL BLADDER SYNDROME

Interstitial cystitis (IC) is a chronic condition that affects the bladder and its ability to hold urine. People with IC need to go to the bathroom more often and feel they have not entirely emptied their bladder after urinating. There is also pressure and pain in the abdominal area associated with IC. Ninety percent of people suffering from IC are women. There is no known specific cause for IC; however, certain beverages and foods like coffee, alcohol, and citrus can irritate the bladder. A specialty within the field of physical therapy is called orthopedic pelvic floor therapy and Thiele massage, which provide both intravaginal and external massage.

## ⇒  *Interstitial Cystitis Protocol*  ⬅

Integrate the following protocol with the onset of symptoms and continue as needed.

- Take 600 milligrams aloe vera capsules 3 times a day.
- Take 1,000 milligrams evening primrose oil 2 times a day.
- Drink 1 to 2 cups of cleavers tea a day.
- Take 1 to 2 kava capsules (each containing 60 milligrams of kavalactones) as needed for pain.
- Gently rub CBD oil over the belly above the bladder twice a day to provide pain relief and relax the musculature.

## URINARY INCONTINENCE

Urinary incontinence is a lack of bladder control. It can range from mild (occasionally leaking urine when straining) to severe (needing to empty the bladder very suddenly and strongly). It commonly occurs as a symptom during pregnancy, after childbirth, or during menopause.

&#8594;&#8594;  *Bladder Support Tea*  &#8592;&#8592;

This tea provides support for bladder symptoms, including UTI, IC, and urinary incontinence.

**MAKES ¾ CUP, ABOUT 36 SERVINGS**

| | |
|---|---|
| 1 ounce lady's mantle | 1 ounce partridgeberry |
| 1 ounce gotu kola | 1 ounce horsetail |
| 1 ounce St. John's wort | 1 ounce corn silk |

Mix all the ingredients together and store in a glass jar in a dark cupboard. When you're ready to make the tea, add a heaping teaspoon of this blend to 2 cups of boiled water, let infuse for 15 minutes, strain, and drink 1 to 2 times a day.

For an overactive bladder, include herbal antispasmodics like valerian tea or gosha-jinki-gan, a traditional Chinese herbal medicine made from ten different herbs and dosed at 5 grams a day.

## FUNGAL INFECTIONS

Fungal infections are caused when a certain strain of fungi attacks an area of the body. Most affect the skin as a rash, especially in regions like the vagina, groin, and anus where skin is moist; however, more serious cases of fungal infections may affect the lungs and nasal biome. People on antibiotics or who have suppressed immune systems are more prone to fungal infections. Examples of fungal infections are athlete's foot, jock itch, ringworm, and yeast infections.

You can apply tea tree oil to fungal infections, though you may require pharmaceutical grade dimethyl sulfoxide (DMSO) to serve as a carrier to penetrate into nail fungus (onychomycosis) infections.

### YEAST INFECTIONS

Vaginal yeast infections can occur when the candida albicans yeast in the body grows out of control. Stress, pregnancy, excess sugar intake, tight underwear that adds heat and moisture, and sex with a new partner can all contribute to a yeast infection. Lactobacilli help to keep yeast under control, and taking garlic internally or as a suppository can help reduce the yeast. Take a minimum of 10 days to go on a very strict protein, vegetable, and fat diet with no starchy carbohydrates, fruits, or sugars. During this time consume probiotic rich foods and lots of garlic and onions.

Garlic is both antifungal and antibacterial. To treat a vaginal yeast infection peel a clove of garlic and, using a needle, run a thin cotton thread through the garlic and tie a small knot so it is easy to retrieve. At bedtime, gently insert the clove in the vagina, allowing the string to hang out. In the morning, gently tug on the string and throw away the garlic. Repeat for 1 to 3 nights. You may repeat this protocol as often as needed until symptoms subside.

## POLYCYSTIC OVARIAN SYNDROME (PCOS)

PCOS is an endocrine disorder caused by a hormonal imbalance that affects 10 to 18 percent of all women of childbearing age and is the leading cause of infertility. It includes excess androgens and polycystic ovaries and often co-occurs with obesity, diabetes, and insulin resistance. Certain medications can also trigger onset.

Treatment and recovery involve all aspects of health: dietary—including a low glycemic, no-grain regimen—herbal medicines, and exercise. A combination of 30 minutes of resistance training, which improves insulin resistance, and 30 minutes of aerobic exercise should be done 5 days a week.

An effective protocol for PCOS combines anti-inflammatory herbs that lower blood glucose and balance hormones. Dietary changes for PCOS should include elimination of refined sugar and flours and poor-quality fats and emphasize hormone- and pesticide-free organic foods. Herbal medicines with best effects for PCOS are shown in the following list.

### PCOS PROTOCOL

- Take herbs that lower blood glucose and enhance insulin metabolism such as berberine-rich plants, like Oregon grape root or berberine supplements (1,000 milligrams twice a day) and cinnamon (500 milligrams 2 times a day).

- Take at least 1 anti-inflammatory herb such as licorice root tea, once a day.

- Take chasteberry extract with 3 milligrams agnuside (1,000 milligrams a day) to help balance hormones.

- Take tribulus, also called bindii (*Tribulus terrestris*), fruit extract with 40 percent saponins (450 milligrams twice a day or whole root powder at 2 grams a day).

- Take white peony root (5 grams of whole root powder or extract providing 252 milligrams paeoniflorin twice a day).

Follow this protocol for 21 days out of the month, take 7 days off, and begin the protocol again.

One way to organize this protocol is to begin your day with a cup of licorice root tea, and for lunch make a smoothie and add the chasteberry, tribulus, and white peony root into a smoothie of 1 cup of your favorite fresh or frozen berries and 1 cup of nut milk. Then take the berberine and cinnamon supplements with breakfast and lunch.

## ENDOMETRIOSIS

Endometriosis occurs when the inner lining of the uterus grows on other organs, typically around the pelvic region, and sometimes spreading out farther to other organs. Complications arise with the displaced tissue, including scar tissue, severe pain, and fertility problems. In addition to genetic risk factors, there is evidence that hormone disruptors in pesticides and in foods contribute to endometriosis.

Endometriosis is a challenging illness to treat, and it requires a comprehensive program for improving health, including reducing stress and toxic and environmental exposures, detoxification, and exercise. Herbal medicine focuses on improving overall health and decreasing pain with the use of analgesics and antispasmodics. The endocannabinoid system is involved with the experience of pain, and women with endometriosis have been found to have lower levels of cannabinoid receptors in endometrial tissue, suggesting the potential role of cannabis, both CBD- and THC-rich strains. A daily low dose of CBD extract will support the endocannabinoid system. Gentle abdominal massages that enhance lymphatic flow and relaxation, and neurofeedback can also be part of the overall strategy.

> →   *Protocol for Endometriosis*   ←

The herbal protocol is the same as for dysmenorrhea (see page 172); however, for severe pain add 500 milligrams of California poppy in glycerite extract 3 times a day, especially when pain interrupts sleep, and topical and sublingual CBD oil or sublingual THC-rich cannabis oil.

## FIBROIDS

Fibroids are tumors (usually noncancerous) that grow in the uterus. Symptoms can include heavy periods, pelvic pain, frequent urination, lower back pain, and pain during intercourse. The naturopathic physician Dr. Tori Hudson has written extensively about the limited success of natural medicine for treating fibroids, and this has been my clinical experience as well. I have worked with many women using Turksa's formula, high-dose pancreatic enzymes, vitamin D, and liver detoxification. Often fibroids improve with menopause, but sometimes they don't. Engaging in a comprehensive effort is worthwhile, as your overall health along with symptoms will improve and fibroid growth can be limited.

## PREGNANCY

There are a number of herbs that can be used safely during pregnancy, but most should be avoided. It is wise to avoid herb use during the first trimester and consider what herbal compounds may be passed to the infant, either internally or topically, during breastfeeding. Moderate the use of spices during pregnancy and rotate the use of different herbs. Chamomile, ginger, and red raspberry leaf are safe and can help to alleviate morning sickness, calm digestion, and help you relax and sleep. Garlic may be used if you are fighting a cold or for infections. Drinking mineral-rich broths with nettles and beet greens provides an easily assimilated source of iron.

### BIRTHING: BREECH POSITION

Moxibustion using mugwort (*Artemisia vulgaris*) applied to the bladder meridian on point BL67 will often facilitate the repositioning of a breeched fetus. Work with an acupuncturist to locate the point, which is the outside corner of the pinky toenail. In this treatment, a moxa stick is held 2 inches from the skin at that point on each foot for 10 to 20 minutes a day for 10 days. Once the baby turns, continue the treatment 3 times a week for 10 minutes during the following week. If labor is delayed or is difficult, this point may be treated again with moxa.

## LACTATION

Lactation can feel overwhelming at times for new moms. Many women worry that they won't produce enough milk to properly nourish their children or have issues with pain. Challenges that may arise during breastfeeding include difficulties in the infant latching, breast engorgement, clogged milk ducts, and mastitis. Clogged milk ducts may occur as pockets of hardness in the breast, and a warm compress can provide relief. Some engorgement will occur with most new breastfeeding mothers, but it is important to nurse your baby frequently and drain your breasts to avoid complications. If left untreated, engorgement or clogged milk ducts can lead to mastitis, an infection of the breast. There are many ways of improving breast milk supply, including the use of herbal galactagogues.

⇥ *Lactation Support Tea* ⇤

Alternate fenugreek seed tea (page 74) and Café de Capomo (page 61) to support milk flow.

## POSTPARTUM

After giving birth, indigenous women in rural western Mexico traditionally bury the umbilical cord underneath a tree on their land. This ritual symbolizes the planting of roots in the land for their child and in the community and thus reaffirms the child's cultural connections. It is this connection to the land that passes from one generation to the next demonstrating the essence of human culture. The American Indian philosopher Dr. Rudolph Ryser calls our attention to the word *culture* with the root *cult* meaning "worship" and *ure* referring to the "earth," echoing the common refrain among indigenous cultures to worship Mother Earth. Culture links the land and its life-giving benefits to the health and well-being of the family and reinforces daily activities and rhythms of nature in women's lives. Consider a ritual that makes sense for you and your family as you explore rituals in chapter 8 (see pages 237–39).

## → *Postpartum Herbs* ←

It is important to stay hydrated after giving birth. Make a tea of white ash (*Fraxinus americana*) to provide strength. Oat straw tea can also be kept in the fridge and drunk cold or warm.

## → *Postpartum Sitz Bath* ←

A sitz bath is a soothing bath where you sit and immerse yourself up to the lower belly in order to relax and heal the pelvic, anal, perineal, and vaginal tissue. After giving the birth, get the go-ahead from your health provider and utilize a sitz bath for some quiet time to soak and heal while breathing in the magnitude of the new being who has arrived.

**MAKES ABOUT ¾ CUP, ENOUGH FOR ABOUT 4 BATHS**

½ ounce Calendula flowers

½ ounce Lavender flowers

½ ounce Shepherd's purse

½ ounce Plantain leaf

½ ounce Red raspberry leaves

½ ounce Yarrow flowers

½ ounce dried sage

Four 6-inch muslin bags

½ cup gray or pink sea salt or
      Epsom salts

Mix the herbs together in a large bowl, fill the muslin bags with the mixture, and tie the strings to close the bags. Soak all the herb-filled bags in 2 quarts of boiled water for 1 hour to make a strong infusion. Remove the bags and add the infusion along with the salt to a bathtub. Alternatively, you can purchase a large plastic or metal tub large enough to sit in comfortably. Add enough additional warm water so that the hips and lower belly are covered and soak for 20 to 30 minutes. You can leave this infusion in the tub for up to 4 baths, and it's helpful to repeat your sitz bath twice a day. Some women find cooler water soothing, so you might do 1 warm and 1 cool bath a day.

**CAUTION:** If you had a cesarean section do not immerse yourself fully or let the wound get wet.

## ⇸ Ashwagandha Bala (Sida cordifolia) Massage Oil ⇷

Make this oil at least 8 weeks in advance of the mother's due date. When the new mother is ready, gently warm the oil and apply to any area she chooses for a soothing postpartum massage. *Bala* means "giving strength" and also "child" in Sanskrit, and this massage oil will help rejuvenate the mother as she nurses her new infant.

**MAKES ABOUT 3 CUPS**

⅔ cup bala root

2 cups organic cold-pressed sesame oil

⅔ cup ashwagandha root

Coarsely chop the herb roots and put them in a pint jar, pressing them to the bottom. Cover over with sesame oil, screw the lid on tightly, and place on a shelf or on your baby altar. After about 8 weeks, strain through a fine cloth and pour into a clean bottle, adding a label with the ingredients and date. If you cannot find bala root, you may use 2 heaping tablespoons of bala root powder instead of the root.

---

**Postpartum Depression and Anxiety**

Postpartum depression and anxiety is a common condition following the birth of a child. It is characterized by feelings of disconnection, challenges with bonding, overwhelming worry, doubt, fear, sorrow, rage, worthlessness, and even suicidality. The drastic drop in estrogen and progesterone after childbirth contributes to mood changes, which are aggravated by the sleep deprivation associated with caring for a newborn infant. Fatigue and worry are normal for new mothers, but postpartum depression and anxiety are diagnosed when these feelings interfere with interpersonal relationships and the mother's ability to care for her child.

There is some evidence that a low level of vitamin D antepartum is a risk factor in postpartum depression, suggesting both sun exposure and supplemental vitamin D are important. Physical exercise antepartum also reduces the risk of depression. Fatigue is a risk factor for depression for two years postpartum, which suggests that having extended family and friends provide childcare and household relief is beneficial.

Herbal remedies for depression and anxiety should be carefully considered if the mother is nursing and could pass herbal constituents to the infant through breast milk. During this "fourth trimester," she should continue to work closely with her health team to get support and advice and consider integrating the following protocol, tailored to her specific needs. While there is extensive prescribing of SSRIs for postpartum depression, it is preferable to instead use standardized herbal teas or tinctures if possible. What is essential is to treat the depression and anxiety in order to safeguard the well-being of mother and infant. This may include bioidentical hormones and psychotherapy and herbs that stabilize or boost mood and reduce anxiety. You may select from chamomile, ashwagandha, oat straw, lemon balm, vervain, hops, or motherwort, all of which are safe while breastfeeding. These herbs are complemented by the use of vitamin D or B complex with minerals, omega-3 fatty acids (rich in DHA), bright-light therapy, massage therapy, reflexology, acupuncture, abdominal hot packs, and sitz baths.

## BREAST HEALTH

Breasts are made up of fatty tissue that covers ducts biologically designed to produce, store, and deliver milk to offspring. Breasts, in particular nipples, are also an important erogenous zone. Breasts may provide nourishment to newborns, swell during menstrual cycle, be painful and lumpy, develop cancer, or be surgically enlarged, reduced, or removed for medical reasons. Breasts benefit from our attention and care. Feel your breast regularly, noting areas of discomfort, lumps, or congestion. Self massage, skin brushing, and lightening up on the brassieres all help to keep lymph flowing and are acts of loving self-care.

Breast cancer affects women at the highest rates in Australia and New Zealand, Europe, and North America and the lowest rates in Africa and Asia. In the United States, about one in eight women develop invasive breast cancer. Women with breast cancer may undergo partial or complete mastectomies and lymph node removal around the breast and underarms. Some women choose to have preventative mastectomies if they carry a genetic risk of breast cancer. The BRCA1 and BRCA2 genetic mutations confer an approximate risk of 70 percent of developing invasive breast cancer, however, less than 10 percent of all breast cancers are due to these mutations. Mammography, a special breast X-ray, is often heralded as an effective cancer screening but is also the subject of controversy since research shows that routine mammography screening does not reduce the rate of late-stage cancer or decrease cancer mortality rates. Mammograms increase exposure to radiation, which for some women increases their risk of cancer, and mammography often finds in situ cancers that result in unnecessary treatment. As in all aspects of health care one benefits from making an informed choice for diagnosis and self-care based on their personal needs.

In many societies, including Western cultures, women and breasts are sexually objectified and this can lead to women's internalization of either positive or negative feelings about their breasts. Women may respond by having elective surgery to enlarge or decrease size. Many smaller women with larger breasts also have surgery to decrease breast size and reduce ergonomic strain that contributes to chronic neck and back pain. Transgender individuals may elect to have breast reduction or enlargement surgeries to align with their gender identity.

## NURSING AND PAINFUL NIPPLES

Our breasts always benefit from massage with warm oil; it is relaxing and allows us to feel for lumps, relax swelling and move lymph along, and reduce pain. Massage also helps milk to flow or soothes painful nipples when we are nursing. It has been shown to decrease pain and prevent engorgement and mastitis.

CAUTION: If using compresses or oils when nursing, make sure you remove the herbal oil from the nipple area prior to nursing.

---

### ⇻ *Poke Root Massage Oil* ⇺

Poke root (*Phytolacca americana*) oil can be massaged into the breasts and around the nipples to ease painful breasts due to lumpiness, mastitis, or clogged milk ducts. Poke root is especially useful if you feel an infection starting.

CAUTION: Poke root can be toxic and should only be used under the guidance of a skilled herbalist or midwife.

---

### ⇻ *Calendula Sweet Almond Breast Massage Oil* ⇺

This oil is soothing for nursing mothers with sore or cracked nipples and prevents and heals chapped skin on your infant. It can also be used by women with fibrocystic breasts, and it is a soothing remedy to wounded tissue and lymph glands after breast surgery.

The oil can be purchased, or it can be made at home as follows: Heat a cup of sweet almond oil on low and gently mix in ½ cup of calendula flowers. Simmer for 1 hour then strain, cool, and bottle. When you want to use the oil, place the bottle in a hot water bath to warm it. Alternatively, you can place the same mixture of flower petals and oil in an amber bottle and put it in a sunny window for 1 month, shaking daily. Then strain and bottle.

CAUTION: If nursing, make sure that you only apply the oil between feedings and that you wash with warm water before nursing, or do not use oil in the nipple area.

## MASTECTOMIES

Following mastectomies many women suffer from pain, loss of range of motion, and lymphedema. They are told that they should feel fine but often do not. As a clinician, I have provided gentle breast, chest, and lymphatic massage to numerous women to reduce their discomfort after mastectomies. This type of massage can be done by a professional; however, a simple massage of tissue can start the healing process. Using one of the oils from page 33, gently and intuitively massage the tissues with one hand, starting from underneath the underarm. Then move both hands to contact the outer perimeter of the breast and slowly stroke lightly toward the nipple.

## FIBROCYSTIC BREAST

Reducing or eliminating underwire bras lessens pressure on delicate lymph nodes. Reduce breast congestion by using an all-natural bristle skin brush and gently brush underneath the underarm toward the heart, including the chest and breast. When you brush the breast do so gently and brush toward the nipple. Coffee enemas and herbs like dandelion and milk thistle enhance the ability of the liver to help excrete estrogen, which contributes to fibrocystic breasts. The Happy Liver Smoothie on page 85 will also aid liver health as will cutting down or eliminating coffee, hard alcohol, and chocolate.

# PERIMENOPAUSE

Perimenopause marks the time when our estrogen and progesterone levels begin to drop, causing irregular periods, hot flashes, vaginal dryness, sleep problems, and mood swings. Oftentimes, perimenopause is more symptomatic than the onset of menopause. Women who have struggled with PMS or painful menses or experienced chronic stress may have more challenging symptoms during perimenopause and menopause. As estrogen and progesterone levels drop, the skin produces less collagen, causing skin to thin and bruise more easily. Increasing rutin-rich herbs like elderberry flower tea and black and green tea and fruits like figs and apples helps reduce bruising.

---

### ⇥ *Perimenopause Smoothie* ⇐

Camu camu (*Myrciaria dubia*) is a versatile berry, with its pulp, seeds, and skin providing antioxidant rich vitamins and minerals. When combined with ginseng, royal jelly, and hops it helps balance the symptoms of perimenopause.

**MAKES 1 SERVING**

6 ounces almond milk

½ cup berries

1 teaspoon evening primrose oil

1 teaspoon camu camu powder

10 drops hops extract

1 small bottle or capsule Korean

    ginseng and royal jelly extract

    (see note)

Add all of the ingredients to a blender and blend until combined. Drink daily for at least 3 months to experience benefits.

**NOTE:** There is a product called Royal 3 Woman's formula by Tang Health Aid that provides capsules as an option instead of liquid ginseng and jelly.

---

## MENOPAUSE

The physical symptoms associated with menopause include hot flashes and chills, insomnia, mood changes, slower metabolism, thinning hair, dry skin, night sweats, and vaginal dryness. Loss of bone density (osteoporosis) is common in the first few years after menopause. Emotionally, one may feel irritable, anxious, depressed, and moody. Many of the changes that begin in perimenopause can become more evident, but for some women menopause is actually easier than perimenopause.

Mother nature has given us many herbs rich in constituents that ease symptoms of menopause and are protective of cognitive function, bone health, and emotional balance. While herbal medicines are important, in my clinical experience many women benefit from bioidentical hormone replacement beginning with progesterone and dehydroepiandrosterone (DHEA) during perimenopause and adding in estrogen and testosterone with the onset of menopause as these will synergize the effects of herbs. One should never use synthetic hormones but should always obtain bioidentical hormones from a compounding pharmacy. Start with adaptogens to manage vasomotor symptoms. Enhancing hormones, ensuring sleep, and regulating moods are central to weathering changes. Continue with the perimenopause smoothie (above) and add in the following menopause brew.

> ### ⇥ *Menopause Brew* ⇤
>
> **MAKES 2 SERVINGS**
>
> Gently simmer a thumb of fresh ginger and 1 teaspoon of fenugreek seeds in 2½ cups of boiling water for 20 minutes. Add 1 teaspoon of St John's wort and 1 teaspoon of sage and let the mixture infuse for 20 more minutes. Strain and drink up to 2 cups daily.

# BONE HEALTH

Our bones are alive! They are made up of mostly calcium and collagen, and while we often take them for granted or think of them as set in place, they are undergoing continuous remodeling as bone cells die and are replaced. When we are younger, bone creation exceeds bone loss and as we age the opposite occurs. Bones and our soft tissue—muscles ligaments and tendons—work closely together. When muscles or ligaments get too tight or too loose bones may not hold their position, leading to pain and excessive wear and tear. Massage and cranial osteopathy are among the many manual therapies that speak the language of bones to help return us to balance.

## OSTEOPOROSIS

Osteoporosis is a condition where the normal balance between the cells that create bone and those that break it down becomes imbalanced, leading to bone loss and lack of new bone formation. It is considered a multi-system with multiple risk factors. Most often, women over 50 are at greatest risk as estrogen and testosterone levels decrease. Additional risk factors include excessive alcohol use, low calcium intake and/or absorption, a history of sedentism, the use of SSRIs (antidepressants), blood thinners like Coumadin, and corticosteroids.

> ### ⇥ *Osteoporosis Prevention Protocol* ⇤
>
> - To strengthen bones, begin by walking and lifting weights and gradually add some soup cans or books to a backpack to wear while walking.
> - Engage in weight-bearing, muscle-strengthening, core-strengthening, and balancing exercises 3 to 5 days a week to prevent falls.
> - Eat dark leafy greens rich in magnesium, calcium, and vitamins K1 and K2.

- Eat bone and vegetable broths and berberine-rich plants to boost bone building activity in the body.

- Supplement with vitamins A, D, E, and K liquid drops.

- Apply bioidentical hormones, especially estrogen and DHEA cream, to vaginal tissue.

- Rotate use of estrogenic herbs in your diet like hops, damiana, licorice, and evening primrose.

- Keep blood sugar levels in normal range.

CAUTION: Be careful about taking too high a dose of calcium supplementation; it doesn't always help and can cause side effects in heart and kidney health. Sometimes you have plenty of circulating calcium—the problem is driving it into the bone, in which case supplementing with minerals such as phosphorous, boron, and strontium is helpful.

---

### ⇒ *Bone Health Smoothie* ⇐

Red sage and horny goat weed (*Epimedium*; *Epimedium sagittatum*) are combined in Chinese Medicine formulas to treat osteoporosis. You can also combine them yourself in the following smoothie recipe, which uses calcium-rich almond milk.

**MAKES 1 SERVING**

1½ cups almond milk

2 heaping tablespoons collagen powder

1 tablespoon whey powder

2 tablespoons horny goat weed powder

20 drops red sage extract

1 teaspoon raw local honey

Add all the ingredients to a blender and blend until combined. Drink daily.

---

## OSTEOARTHRITIS

Osteoarthritis is most common in women and risk and disability increase with age. Finding effective alternatives to NSAIDs is essential to avoid dangerous side effects of these drugs. Alternatives include the use of NF-kB inhibitor herbs, including turmeric, boswellia, green tea, and resveratrol. Anti-inflammatory lubricants, including evening primrose oil and collagen, provide nourishment to the joints. There is a connection between diabetes and arthritis as they both arise from inflammation; hence blood glucose management is also good osteoarthritis prevention. Injections of hyaluronic acid are safe and naturally supportive of some joints, especially the knees. This treatment reduces pain so exercise can strengthen the muscles around the affected joints.

# HEALTHY SKIN

Skin is our largest organ—a road map to what is going on inside our body. It is an important organ of detoxification. When toxins, allergies, hormones, nutritional deficiencies, and emotional stress are released through the skin, they tell their story in pimples, boils, acne, itchy bumps, fungus, eczema, psoriasis, and more. Healthy skin begins with nourishing ourselves on the inside, reducing exposure to toxins, and then helping our skin to effectively release the waste. One of the best ways to support skin health is to sweat, in dry or moist heat and through exercise, and to moisturize within with borage oil and on the skin itself with coconut oil.

## SKIN AND FACIAL REJUVENATION

Caring for the facial skin can be a profound act of self-care; this is the face we share with the world, and the brightness of the skin and the eyes convey our connection to others and to our deep vitality. Exposure to ultraviolet rays or environmental toxins, smoking nicotine, drinking too much alcohol, or eating a lot of sugar will decrease the ability of our skin to do its job: insulate and protect our inner organs, regulate our body temperature, dispose of waste, and facilitate our sensory life, mediating between the inner and outer worlds.

We will all wrinkle and droop, spot, and fade as our skin dries and collagen and hormones decrease. This process accelerates at menopause. But our skin, when treated properly, is the well-earned map of our lives telling our story through the scars, stretch marks, and our heritage and genetics. To celebrate this personal map, I have created this simple facial rejuvenation oil that complements all the inner rejuvenation methods you use to support your vital energy. Hydration, inside and out, is essential. If you use bioidentical hormone creams you can also apply them every other day to the facial skin, rotating with vaginal application. Apply estrogen in the morning and progesterone in the evening.

## ⇸ *Topical Facial Rejuvenation Oil* ⇐

**MAKES 5 APPLICATIONS**

¼ cup sesame oil

20 drops pure hyaluronic acid serum

10 drops damask rose oil

2 vitamin E oil capsules (400 IU each of mixed tocopherols and tocotrienols)

Add all the ingredients together in a small ceramic container and mix well. Apply a thin layer to the skin before bed every night for 5 days or as long as the mixture lasts. This mixture should be kept in the fridge and made fresh each week.

## ⇸ *Using a Kansa Wand and Marma Point Massage* ⇐

Obtain a small kansa wand for face or foot massage. Apply the facial rejuvenation oil and then use the wand to apply gentle pressure to stress points on the face, including the marma points. Stress points are areas where stress collects on the face, often under the eyes, sinus points, the forehead, jaw, and smile lines. Marma points are subtle energy points, similar to acupuncture points, that when released relax the face and have a beneficial effect on vitality and well-being throughout the body. Facial massage is always performed by making circles in a clockwise direction as you move down the face and neck in the direction of the lymphatic flow toward the heart. This action also helps ease jaw tension and can become part of your daily self-care routine. I like to use the kansa wand and facial massage after I do skin brushing each evening.

## ⇸ *Green Tea Facial Mask* ⇐

Soak 2 chamomile or black tea bags in warm water ahead of time and put them in the freezer for 10 minutes.

Then make a green tea mask by adding ¼ teaspoon of green tea powder to ½ cup of freshly ground flaxseed. Beat an egg and add it to the powder and seed to make a paste. Apply the mask to the face and then apply the cold tea bags over the eyes. Lie down for 20 to 45 minutes and then discard the tea bags and rinse the mask off with warm water.

## → Skin-So-Smoothie ←

This smoothie supports skin health from the inside out, improving elasticity and increasing vitality.

**MAKES 1 TO 2 SERVINGS**

2 cups cold tea made with ½ teaspoon green tea powder

2 to 4 tablespoons (10 to 20 grams) collagen peptides

1 cup fresh or frozen berries

200 milligrams hyaluronic acid powder

10 drops burdock root powder

10 drops gotu kola extract

1,000 grams amla (Indian gooseberry) powder

1,000 milligrams vitamin C powder (with rutin)

1 teaspoon raw local honey or 10 drops stevia

Chamomile Tea Ice Cubes (page 117, optional)

Add all the ingredients to a blender and blend until combined. You can add chamomile tea ice cubes if desired. Drink daily for at least 8 weeks to notice improvement.

# SEXUAL HEALTH

As we grow and change so does our expression of our sexuality. How we feel at the start of puberty may be very different from how we feel after being in a long-term relationship, at the end of a seventy-hour work week, having spent years in retreat alone or celibate, after giving birth, or at menopause. If we have been wounded sexually as children or adults, our sexual expression can be fraught and will benefit from proactive healing through verbal or somatic therapies. Whatever our stage of life, our sexuality is ours to claim, assert, and renew as we decide.

Sexual problems affect up to 45 percent of women at some point in their lives and can include a loss of interest in sex, the inability to feel satisfied or have orgasms, or the inability to say no to sex. Women may question their sexuality or who they want to have as their partner, or they may feel oppressed by negative religious or family beliefs. Stress and anxiety are major factors that affect sexual health and in turn affect intimate relationships and contribute to low self-esteem, causing further stress. Supporting the nervous system is the foundation for supporting sexual well-being, and connecting with other women to share experiences, feelings, and ideas can reduce isolation and start the healing process.

# LIBIDO

*Libido* is another term for our sex drive. There are many physical, emotional, and mental influences on our libido, and even religious beliefs and experiences can affect it. Low libido affects women of all ages and is on the rise because our lives can be so full and stressful. It can be caused by chronic stress, work/life imbalances, and interpersonal conflicts with your partner. Among women with a history of sexual assault, there may be a trigger at any point in life during which memories reemerge and affect libido. Thus, just because you have "dealt with it" doesn't mean that a new layer of physical or emotional distress cannot emerge and ask to be addressed. If this occurs, listen deeply to your body and mind; these messages really need to be addressed before energy can continue to flow to libido.

Medications that can dampen libido include antidepressants, beta-blockers used for high blood pressure, and estrogen blockers used in cancer treatment. Use the herbal remedies in this book and work with a professional to find alternatives to these medications. Sedentariness can dampen libido as it exacerbates dissociation; just feeling out of our bodies and out of touch with ourselves and our needs can dampen our drive, so get out and move. Libido can drop at menopause; however, bioidentical hormones and the following herbal protocols will bring the zing back into your zazz.

## LOW LIBIDO? FEELING FOGGY?

One quick fix for a dragging libido is to take 400 milligrams of Korean ginseng 2 to 3 times a day. Another is to drink the delicious Chocolate Walnut Banana Libido Smoothie (recipe follows). All of these ingredients work together synergistically to enhance libido, balance hormones and brain neurotransmitters, and support adrenal function while enhancing relaxation.

### ⇥ *Chocolate Walnut Banana Libido Smoothie* ⇤

**MAKES 1 SERVING**

1 cup oat milk

½ frozen banana

¼ cup raw walnuts

1 to 2 tablespoons maca root powder

1 to 2 tablespoons cocoa powder

2,000 milligrams evening primrose oil

Damiana extract (or add 2 tablespoons strong infusion and omit 2 tablespoons oat milk)

1,000 milligrams horny goat weed
  extract or 100 milligrams icariin
  supplement

Add all the ingredients to a blender and blend until combined. Drink daily for 3 months.

# PAINFUL VAGINAL SEX

Vaginal pain can occur upon penetration for a variety of physical, structural, or emotional reasons. A previous history of sexual abuse, pelvic tension due to religious teachings, fear of pregnancy, chronic vaginal infections that have upset the balance of flora and lubrication, and endometriosis can all contribute to pain. Pain can also occur at menopause when low estrogen leads to drying and thinning of the vaginal walls. Working with a clinician is important to identify the cause. If you have ruled out structural or medical problems, physical therapy specialists have training in releasing pelvic floor tension with biofeedback or manual therapies that can retrain constricted musculature. It can also be helpful to purchase a silicone sex toy to use on your own with lots of lubricant to explore the penetration process and learn to release muscle tension slowly and gently.

## LUBRICATION AT ALL AGES

If dryness is your issue, use an integrated approach to enhance vaginal lubrication by combining internal and external lubricants. See the following lube suggestions for effective treatments.

### → *External Vaginal Lube* ←

Pierce a 400 IU vitamin E (edible oil mixed tocopherols and tocotrienols) capsule and gently rub it along the vaginal walls daily.

If menopausal, obtain bioidentical estrogen and apply it 3 times a week to the vaginal walls. Natural hormone experts suggest applying bioidentical hormone creams, such as progesterone, estrogen (Biest), testosterone, and DHEA to the vaginal tissue for maximum absorption and effect.

### ⇒ *Lubricate the Vagina with Foods* ⇐

Two easy internal treatments for reducing dryness are (1) take 1 to 3 grams of evening primrose oil a day and (2) add 2,000 milligrams of maca powder to any of your smoothies. A shatavari ghee lubricant can also be of help for lubrication and vaginal health and can be purchased or made at home. To make the lubricant, add 2 ounces of shatavari powder to 1 quart of simmering water. Simmer until reduced by ¾ and then strain out the herb powder. Pour the infusion back into the pan, add 1 cup of ghee, and simmer until the liquid is absorbed. Cool and bottle. Keep in the fridge to add on top of steamed vegetables. If you want a touch of sweetness, add a drop of stevia to it while it melts on your food.

# THRIVING THROUGH SURGERY

Sometimes we cannot avoid surgery, and other times we may choose it for a variety of reasons, including gender affirmation. Herbs can be used to prepare the body before surgery and aid in its recovery after. Any herbal regimen should be stopped at least 3 days prior to surgery to avoid any interactions with any medication being administered, and herbs with blood-thinning effects should be stopped at least a week prior to surgery and for at least 3 days afterward. Herbs on this list include (but are not limited to) garlic, ginkgo, willow, meadowsweet, and St. John's wort. Forgoing alcohol for a few weeks prior to and after surgery is also recommended since it has a blood-thinning effect and disrupts the healing process. It is advisable to work with an herbal professional who knows the risks related to the use of herbs in conjunction with surgery. Someone familiar with your body and the type of procedure you are undergoing can help to build an herbal regimen that is most supportive to you as an individual.

## HERBS FOR PRESURGICAL PREPARATION

Some herbs that may be useful when preparing for surgery include those that activate the immune system, such as reishi and shiitake mushrooms. Shiitake is especially easy to add to the diet whether fresh or dried; try a handful in your omelet or veggie stir-fry!

Milk thistle also supports the body both pre- and post-surgery by preparing and protecting your liver from the effects of drugs administered through the process. When your liver is getting help to detoxify, the effects of anesthesia can be lessened post-surgery. Add 15 grams of ground seed to your daily smoothie! Alternatively, a standardized extract can be used.

Contemplating and going through surgery is stressful. Use an adaptogen for the month prior to enhance your resilience and then also during your recovery.

## HERBS FOR POST-SURGERY RECOVERY

Allow yourself to sleep following surgery; sleep is the body's way of restoring balance. Use the adaptogens for stress relief until midday and then use nervines in the afternoons to help you rest.

After surgery, herbs can be wonderful allies throughout the healing process. Topically, a salve of comfrey and arnica can be used on bruised tissue (not on open wounds). Homeopathic arnica tablets can be taken internally as well. St. John's wort, calendula, plantain, and yarrow can all be used in salves, balms, or sitz baths (recipe follows) as vulneraries, to aid in tissue healing.

### ⇥ *Calendula and Plantain Sitz Bath* ⇤

Whether you are going through gender affirmation surgery or recovering from childbirth, a calendula and plantain sitz bath will help heal the genitourinary region. Steep a large handful of calendula flowers and plantain in 1 to 2 quarts of boiling water and allow to sit, covered, for up to 2 hours. Strain the liquid into a shallow bath or tub and add more warm water until desired depth is achieved (enough to comfortably sit in). This will help to heal and soothe irritated tissue. If you don't have a bathtub, a large plastic or metal washtub can do the trick. Add a soft waterproof rubber or plastic pillow to ease sitting. If you have had chest or breast surgery, a poultice of this mixture can be applied to the wound areas.

## HERB, SPICE, AND FOOD COMBINATIONS AFTER SURGERY

The following herbs and spices can be of great help for recovering after surgery:

- Take 15 milliliters daily of milky oats tincture or glycerite during the first week of recovery to help rebuild the nervous system after surgery.

- Turmeric powder added to your spice mixes and recipes can help reduce inflammation.

- Bone broths infused with herbs like burdock, dandelion, garlic, turmeric, and ginger can move toxins out of the body, decrease inflammation, help rebuild tissue, and support healthy digestion.

- Mustard seed, cinnamon, and cayenne sprinkled on food increase circulation and promote healing.

- Chocolate brings pleasure to body and mind, and it speeds recovery of inflamed tissue.

# CHILDREN: SPECIAL CONCERNS

All symptoms tell a story and this is especially true with children who may not have the language to express their distress. While physical symptoms may be easier to describe, children may not understand why they feel anxious or depressed or cannot concentrate. Here I explore a few health challenges infants and children commonly experience that respond well to herbal interventions. Some herbs are contraindicated for children, and you will want to check any herb before you use it; however, the majority of herbs will be safe.

## SAFE HERBS FOR CHILDREN

The following is a list of the herbs that are safe for children:

- Mint or cinnamon tea soothe a bellyache or diarrhea.

- Thyme and fenugreek tea help reduce and move gas.

- Garlic and echinacea can prevent or reduce symptoms of a cold or infection.

- Chamomile (unless the child has a ragweed allergy), lavender oil aromatherapy, or lavender flowers can be put in pillows to aid sleep.

- Lemon balm, California poppy, and calendula salve soothe boo-boos and diaper rash.

- Honey and lemon soothe a sore throat.

- Clove oil applied to a toothache helps dull the pain.

- Cayenne pepper stops bleeding when applied to the wound (including a nose bleed).

- Licorice root (small amount) with horehound or elderberry in a cough syrup or candied lozenges reduce respiratory discomfort.

You may also use herbs in baths, poultices, or as topical applications, which are very safe and effective delivery methods to use for children.

### CLARK'S RULE FOR ADJUSTING HERBAL MEDICINE DOSAGE FOR CHILDREN BETWEEN AGES 2 AND 18

There are several formulas, including Clark's, Dilling's, and Young's, for adjusting dose based on age or weight. I prefer Clark's Rule, which is based on weight and is determined as follows: Divide the child's weight (in pounds) by 150, then give the child that fraction of the adult dose as the appropriate child's dose. For example, for a 50-pound child give 50/150 (or ⅓) of the adult dose. Thus if the adult dose is 30 drops of a glycerite taken 3 times a day, the child's dose will be 10 drops taken 3 times a day.

## COLDS, FLU, BRONCHITIS, PNEUMONIA

The recipe for *Caliente Curación* on page 48 is an old-timey remedy and this recipe is a way to adapt it to make popsicles that children can suck on when they are fighting a cold, flu, bronchitis, or pneumonia.

## ⇻ Children's Caliente Popsicles for a Sore Throat ⇷

**MAKES 4 POPSICLES**

Sometimes children are hesitant to take fire cider, and yet it is just the perfect medicine for a sore throat or cold. These popsicles make it easier for them to swallow it.

Simmer 1 tablespoon of slippery elm bark powder in 6 ounces of mango or pineapple juice for 15 minutes. Strain, then add to 6 ounces of *Caliente Curación* (see page 48) mix, and then pour into a BPA-free, 3-ounce popsicle mold and freeze.

For a variation on this recipe, use licorice root instead of slippery elm bark and chicken broth instead of juice and follow the recipe. You can also add some coconut milk and honey to sweeten the mix before you freeze it.

## ⇻ Mustard Seed Poultice ⇷

**MAKES 1 TO 2 POULTICES**

1 cup flaxseed (freshly ground or
    purchased as flaxseed meal)
1 tablespoon mustard seed (freshly
    ground or purchased as ground
    mustard or powder)

¼ cup water
1 tablespoon virgin cold-pressed
    olive oil
Hot water bottle

Carefully add the ground mustard to the flaxseed meal in a large bowl. Gently stir in the water to make a thick paste. The paste should hold together and not be runny.

Place the ill child in bed so that their head and chest are slightly elevated. Rub olive oil generously from the neck, down the chest, and all the way to the beginning of the belly.

With your fingers, gently apply a thin layer of paste about 1 inch thick, starting at the bottom of the neck, at the clavicles, and make a rectangle of paste all the way down to the diaphragm. Make sure you apply the paste only to the skin that is covered with olive oil. The mustard is a rubefacient, and the olive oil will protect the skin from irritation. When the plaster is placed, put a plastic bag over it, then a towel, then a hot water bottle over the chest, and cover it all with two blankets.

Let sit for 1 hour, occasionally checking on the patient to make sure the skin is not burning or too hot. At the end of an hour use the plastic to gather up the plaster. It can be discarded or saved and used the next day. Remove the remaining plaster and olive oil with a warm damp cloth and keep the patient warm.

The patient may now drink a cup of Ayurvedic Polarity Tea (see page 42) or if they are hungry they can eat some plain chicken broth with lemon, garlic, and onion. The plaster can be repeated daily as needed.

---

## ASTHMA

Allergens, air pollution, and exercise can all contribute to asthma. The hyperventilation of asthma leads to anxiety and alters blood gases, which in turn exacerbates asthma and anxiety. Many children with asthma are allergic to foods, especially the lactose in bovine dairy, which also creates a lot of mucus. Eliminating dairy and pro-inflammatory foods like sugar and white flour and eating acidic foods such as animal protein and bone broths can help. There is also evidence that a probiotic rich diet also helps asthma.

Apple cider vinegar baths can also be effective. Add 1 cup of white or apple cider vinegar to a bath and soak for 20 minutes a day. You can also place an air purifier in the bedroom and run it all day with the windows closed and then turn it off during sleep time, unless the white noise is a comfort. Another very effective approach to reducing airway constriction is to apply a cold ice pack to the middle of the spine between the shoulder blades for 15 minutes a day.

Herbal medicines are especially effective for asthma and can be used in extracts in between meals. These include khella (*Ammi visnaga*), Chinese skullcap (*Scutellaria baicalensis*), and astragalus. A magnesium-rich diet is also very important for asthma, and taking a nightly warm (not hot) Epsom salt bath in which a few drops of lavender essential oil have been added can be helpful. If a child is sensitive to seasonal pollens and grasses, remove clothing upon entering the house from outside, take a shower, and rinse the nostrils and sinuses with a saline spray or a neti pot (a small ceramic container that allows for easy nasal irrigation with a saline solution).

### ⟩⟩  *Asthma Mocha Smoothie (Hot or Cold)*  ⟨⟨

This hot mocha can also be made as an iced smoothie. Drink it for breakfast, lunch, or a snack but not after 3:00 PM. This smoothie is anti-inflammatory and an adaptogen that also eases breathing, as both chocolate and coffee open airways. Depending on the age of the child you might eliminate or reduce the coffee. However, if this smoothie allows you to reduce the use of steroidal inhalers then the coffee should not be a problem. Just don't combine coffee and steroids. This recipe can be used by anyone weighing 130 pounds or more. If weighing less, take this recipe in divided doses and adjust the herbal medicine amounts up or down as needed depending on the child's weight.

**MAKES 1 SERVING (SEE HEADNOTE)**

1 cup hemp milk

1 heaping tablespoon pure cocoa

2 to 4 tablespoons espresso or cold
    brewed or French press coffee

1 teaspoon coconut oil

10 drops khella extract

¼ teaspoon ground ashwagandha
    or 10 drops extract

¼ teaspoon ground turmeric
    or 10 drops extract

¼ teaspoon ground ginger
    or 10 drops extract

Raw local honey or stevia to sweeten

**HOT:** In a small saucepan over low heat, add the espresso and hemp milk, bring to a simmer, and add the cocoa and coconut and whisk until blended. Remove from heat, add the herbal extracts, and mix to combine.

**COLD:** Add all the ingrediends to a blender and blend until combined.

Drink 1 to 2 times a day before 3:00 PM since both coffee and chocolate can be stimulating and interrupt sleep.

---

# BELLYACHES

Bellyache are common in children ages 4 to 8, with the main causes being diet, stress, and growing pains. Constipation, food intolerances, food allergies, diarrhea, and intestinal gas are common causes of bellyaches. In more serious cases, the cause of the bellyache may be an infection or appendicitis.

One easy treatment is to make a chamomile and fennel tea and place a warm pack on the belly and a pillow under the knees. Another is to perform the Bellyache Rock.

## ↠ *Bellyache Rock* ↞

Sometimes a bellyache is a symptom of anxiety. This rocking is a method that you can try when anxiety and a bellyache occur together.

Have the child lie face up with a pillow under the knees and the neck. Place a warm towel over the belly (you can heat up a slightly damp hand towel in the microwave for 3 minutes). Rub some chamomile oil on the belly and, sitting on the right side, place your left hand on the forehead just above the eyebrows and your right hand on the belly, so your little finger borders the pubic bone but does not touch it. Hold the hand on the forehead steady and with your right hand give a very gentle rocking back and forth for a minute, then hold for 30 seconds, letting the warmth and energy from your hand and the towel penetrate, and then rock again. This will alleviate much of the distress. If you feel or hear gas during the rocking this is a good sign as gas can cause belly pain. You may then decide to give a very gentle massage in the direction of peristalsis (clockwise) to the colon to help move the gas along to be released. Following this your child may want a little fennel tea.

---

# EARACHES

Ear infections occur when fluid builds up in the ear, causing inflammation. Children can be reacting to viruses, milk, or airborne allergens. Antibiotics tend to make things worse; the research does not warrant their use, and they cause a cascade of microbiome disruption that can last for years. Better to use this herbal eardrop recipe.

### ⇥ *Herbal Eardrops* ⇤

**MAKES ABOUT ½ CUP**

3 cloves garlic, chopped

½ teaspoon mullein leaf and flowers

½ teaspoon calendula flowers

½ teaspoon St. John's wort

½ cup virgin cold-pressed olive oil

400 IU vitamin E (mixed tocopherols and tocotrienols)

Put the garlic and the herbs in a clean, dry, heatproof canning jar. Fill the jar with oil until the herbs and garlic are completely submerged. If necessary, using a clean utensil, push all plant material to the bottom of the jar to ensure it is fully covered with oil.

Place the covered jar in a slow cooker with a few inches of water, enough to gently warm the jar but not enough to get any water in the oil. Turn the slow cooker onto the lowest setting and allow the herbs to infuse in the oil for at least 1 hour and up to 8 hours. Let the herbal oil cool just enough to handle but not enough that the oil thickens prior to straining. Strain the oil through a piece of cheesecloth to remove any plant materials. It is important to strain carefully as leftover particulates can cause your oil to spoil more quickly. Bottle in a clean, dry dropper bottle and store in the refrigerator.

Warm oil to room temperature prior to use or place the bottle for a minute in a saucepan with boiled water to warm before using. Add 2 drops to the affected ear twice a day until discomfort resolves.

---

## SLEEP ISSUES OF CHILDREN

There are a variety of problems that can interfere with restful, consistent sleep in children at each stage of development. The American Academy of Pediatrics provides the following guidelines for the amount of sleep children require for optimal health every 24 hours.

- Infants 4 to 12 months should sleep 12 to 16 hours

- Children 1 to 2 years—11 to 14 hours

- Children 3 to 5 years—10 to 13 hours

- Children 6 to 12 years—9 to 12 hours

- Teenagers 13 to 18 years—9 to 10 hours

- After age 18 most adults require 8 to 9 hours

Sleep patterns are governed by circadian rhythm, the 24-hour sleep/wake cycle that follows the light and dark of the day. Stress, caffeine, exposure to electronics and light at night, irregular sleep patterns, and sleep-disordered breathing all disrupt this cycle and thus disrupt sleep. Sleep-disordered breathing includes obstructive sleep apnea, snoring, and mouth breathing, all of which affect physical and emotional development.

By grade school half of all children are not getting enough sleep, and by adolescence most teens are not getting enough sleep. Some school systems have made school start times later, recognizing that teens in particular require more sleep than early classes allow. Pre- and perinatal trauma, including a difficult birth, can create stress for the infant and lead to difficulty sleeping. Cesarean births also appear to disrupt sleep patterns, so research suggests the new method called "natural cesarean," which attempts to mirror many of the patterns of a vaginal birth for the mother and child to mitigate these effects. Many mothers and infants benefit from biodynamic cranialsacral therapy before and after birth.

Using herbal medicine to aid sleep begins with diagnosing the problem followed by eliminating the cause(s). A general approach is to combine adaptogens to help cope with stress, nervines and sedatives to relax the nervous system during the evening, and muscle relaxants from magnesium-rich foods and herbs or herbal body soaks. Herbal antihistamines (and air purifiers) if breathing is challenged by sinus or respiratory congestion can also be integrated into the care plan. Here, I address a few specific concerns that affect infant and child sleep.

### NIGHT TERRORS

Night terrors are caused by the overstimulation of the nervous system while asleep. When the body transitions from REM (rapid eye movement) to non-REM sleep, children can experience a spontaneous fear reaction, or night terror. These reactions typically occur 2 to 3 hours after children fall asleep, and children are not aware they are having them. Eighty percent of children who have night terrors have a family member with some sort of sleep disturbance. As the nervous system matures, night terrors become less common.

A hot water bottle (no electric pads), along with a lavender diffuser or sachet or a magnesium sulfate bath before bed, is restful for the nervous system. Rocking and foot massages with chamomile oil before sleep can help too. There is also a special pressure point known as "serene sleep" that is found at the base of the skull just behind the ear, in the soft place where your neck muscles connect to your jawline. Placing your forefinger there with mild pressure for 10 minutes can help to prevent night terrors.

### BED-WETTING

Most bed-wetting in children is genetic; the majority of children who wet their beds have a parent who also wet the bed. Bed-wetting that develops after a child has been continent at night often signals anxiety or sexual abuse, which requires professional consultation. Children outgrow bed-wetting, and the best approach is to reduce anxiety and shame and ensure that skin integrity is maintained so that no rashes develop.

Suo Quan is a Chinese medicine that has been used for bed-wetting and can be purchased at a Chinese Medicine pharmacy. It is a mixture of equal parts black cardamom (*Alpinia oxyphylla*), Chinese yam (*Dioscorea oppositifolia*), and evergreen lindera (*Lindera aggregate*).

## COLIC IN INFANTS

Colic can occur in infants of 2 to 3 or more weeks old, and formula can be a culprit. Here are a few helpful solutions:

- Make a slippery elm bark pudding either from the bark or the powder by gently simmering 2 heaping tablespoons of the bark or powder in 2 cups of water for 20 minutes and then straining. You can store extra "pudding" in the fridge for up to a week and warm for use when required. Use a dropper or your finger to place a drop on the tongue of the infant 3 times a day.

- A combination extract of 18 milligrams chamomile, 130 milligrams lemon balm, and tyndallized *Lactobacillus acidophilus* has been found to be more effective in the treatment of infant colic than standard treatment with simethicone. It is sold commercially as Colimil Baby with a suggested dose of 1 milliliter twice a day.

- Apply a cool towel soaked in strong chamomile tea just below the rib cage.

- A diffuser with lavender helps the infant relax.

## TEETHING

Teeth begin to erupt in babies between 6 months and 2 years. This puts pressure on the gums, inflaming them and causing pain and discomfort. Signs of teething include restlessness, drooling, lack of appetite, increased crying, and biting of objects. This frozen herbal cloth recipe combines a soothing cold cloth to chew on while delivering calming analgesic herbs to aid this important developmental passage with ease.

### ⇻ *Frozen Herbal Cloth for Teething* ⇺

**MAKES 4 TO 6 CLOTH STRIPS**

1 teaspoon whole cloves
2 cups water

3 bags chamomile tea

In a small saucepan over medium heat, simmer the cloves in the water for 20 minutes and then turn off the heat. Add the bags of chamomile tea and let steep. Strain off the cloves and tea and let cool.

Cut a washcloth into 4 to 6 strips, soak the strips in the tea mixture, and place them on a small tray in the freezer. When frozen peel off one at a time and allow your infant to chew on the cloth.

---

## CHILDREN AND MENTAL HEALTH

As a mental health specialist treating children as well as adults I have witnessed a great deal of misdiagnosis of children's mental health. This is mostly due to changing cultural values, along with the latest marketing ploys of pharmaceutical companies. Did you know that during the 1960s, childhood autism was blamed on a cold, uncaring "refrigerator mother"? This absurd idea traumatized and blamed already stressed-out parents and did nothing to improve the health of the child.

Cultural pressures affect teachers, administrators, mental health and primary health providers, and even parents. There is an increasing trend to assign adult diagnostic categories like bipolar disorder and psychosis to children and then give them multiple drugs. This never works, and it often leads to irremediable side effects, including changes in neurological function, often for life.

### ANXIETY

Anxiety in children is a common occurrence. Birth trauma, biology, family, and environment can all contribute to a child's anxiety. Social dynamics at school, the stress of extracurricular performance, and exposure to loss, violence, or trauma all contribute to anxiety. A diet high in refined foods can also affect anxiety. Perinatal nutrition, emphasizing essential fatty acids, including fish as well as gamma linolenic acid (GLA) oils like borage or evening primrose, is essential to brain development of the fetus. Parental stress during pregnancy can be a factor in a child's anxiety, as high levels of stress hormones appear to affect the fetus and the resulting capacity of the child to tolerate stress.

Nothing triggers anxiety faster than a disruption in parental caregiving. Divorce and separation rank high as a cause of anxiety and some learning disorders. However, it cannot always be avoided. Attachment, connection, and safety are physical as well as emotional experiences. Touch, physical movement, and play therapy, along with herbal and nutritional medicine such as chamomile tea, can be combined to reduce anxiety in children.

## » *Chamomile Elixir and Massage Oil* «

Chamomile is also known as "little apple" because of its fragrant apple-like smell. It is a safe herb for kids and adults alike and can be used as an internal or external treatment.

Make a chamomile elixir by concentrating the chamomile by steeping 6 chamomile tea bags in 2 cups of just-boiled water for 1 hour. Strain and store it in the fridge, retaining half as a liquid that can be added to a soup. To the other half, add raw honey to make popsicles or ice cubes.

For external use of chamomile for anxiety, make a massage oil by gently simmering 1 cup of chamomile flowers, fresh or dried, in 1 quart of almond oil for 2 hours and then straining through a muslin or cheesecloth cloth. Use as a topical massage oil for anxiety.

## » *Rocking* «

Rocking can reduce children's anxiety and distress and help them fall asleep. Rocking also reduces anxiety in the person doing the rocking, so everyone will benefit. Rocking synchronizes brain rhythms and increases sleep spindles, which lead to a quicker, more restful sleep.

Have your child lie on their right side. The right side activates the rest cycle of the right brain hemisphere and will induce sleep more quickly. Place a pillow under their neck. Some children also feel comfortable hugging a pillow at their belly. Sit behind the child. Everything that you do in this position should feel easy and natural. Take your left palm, fingers pointed upward at 12 o'clock and place gently but firmly on the sacrum, the triangular bone at the base of the spine, so that the outer edge of the little finger is just above the intergluteal cleft before the buttocks (the hand will not be in contact with the buttocks), and the thumb is around the sacroiliac line (the joint between the sacrum and the ilium bones of the pelvis). In essence, you are covering the sacrum with the palm of your hand. Place your right palm on the back of the neck on the cervical vertebrae and cup your hand gently around the neck. The quality of touch is very light with just a little, soothing pressure. Very gently begin rocking the sacrum by pushing with the left palm. You don't need to get a lot of movement for this to work, and your movement should be adjusted for the comfort of the child. Do this for a minimum of 10 to 20 minutes, with gentle suggestions to close the eyes and breathe more deeply, until the child falls asleep or is sufficiently relaxed.

## SUPPORTING NEURODIVERSITY IN ALL CHILDREN

Neurodiversity is a term of reference applied to people who demonstrate neurological differences and includes many variations in learning and behavior. Some examples include people with attention deficit hyperactivity disorder (ADHD), dyslexia, and Tourette's, as well as people who are on the autism spectrum. The neurodiversity social movement reflects the growing awareness that rather than being defined as disabilities, these are styles of learning and behavior that reflect the creative, adaptive diversity of the human genome and styles of brain-mind function that evolved in response to adaptive needs over millennia. This diversity demands that we adapt and provide innovative opportunities for growth and learning instead of trying to control and suppress the symptoms. Here I address a few of these many important diverse styles with which I have had successful clinical experience.

### ADHD

ADHD describes a behavioral condition marked by inattention, impulsivity, and hyperactivity. Spontaneous behavior is natural in children, but it is often misdiagnosed as ADHD. There is a lot of controversy about this diagnosis among many professionals who suggest it does not even exist. In my clinical practice I find these children are very creative and often have kinesthetic learning styles that are not being addressed in their schools. Stress and trauma, sedentariness, pro-inflammatory foods and food sensitivities, and hypoglycemia often underlie the symptoms of ADHD. Aspartame is a particular problem and should be eliminated.

The nutritional and movement suggestions for anxiety (see pages 205–206) also apply to ADHD since anxiety and ADHD often go together. Martial arts and fencing are ideal activities for these children as well, as they combine movement with body awareness. Look for a nutritional supplement that includes 15 to 20 amino acids in their free form, including but not limited to 5-hydroxytryptophan, L-glutamine, glycine, L-methionine, L-serine, taurine, L-threonine, and L-tyrosine. Chocolate and rhodiola support focus during the day and can be used when transitioning off stimulant medications. A glycerite or tea combining American skullcap, passionflower, and gotu kola supports relaxed attention in the evening.

### AUTISM SPECTRUM

Among my first polarity and cranialsacral patients were young children with a diagnosis of autism. Their therapists brought them to my jungle clinic, and there we prepared healthy gluten- and casein-free meals, drank antioxidant-rich teas, drummed, danced, and engaged in challenging walks in the jungle that required the children to pay close attention lest they fall off the cliff. We used lavender to calm them and went swimming in ice-cold waterfalls, which induces relaxation and body awareness. Upon assessing their energy fields, I found that most often there was a great deal of energy around the head and above but not much in the limbs, hands, and feet. So in addition to lots of rocking, I did hand and foot massage, which was very calming.

The needs of a child on the autism spectrum are diverse, and what helps one may not be helpful to another. The approach to autism using herbs is a nonspecific overall approach that helps optimize all aspects of the child's well-being. This includes improving digestive, endocrine, and immunological health, supporting brain function, including mitochondrial and phospholipid (special fats) communication, and reducing toxic load. There are no easy answers here, but every safe intervention can be applied one step at a time as the child can tolerate.

Nutritionally there is good evidence that many children on the autism spectrum have significant gut and digestive problems that warrant a gluten- and casein-free diet, and food sensitivities should be explored. These children are often sensitive to artificial coloring, flavors, and sweeteners. The brassica vegetables, which are high in glucoraphanin, have been found to reverse oxidative stress and improve mitochondrial function, leading to improved behaviors in children on the autism spectrum. This may best be tolerated as a powder added to a smoothie, 30 milligrams once a day. The nasal spray application using a patented medicine with Borneo camphor, a compound derived from the *Dryobalanops sumatrensis* tree, also showed success at improving children's social skills.

Daily Epsom salt baths with favorite essential oils added to the water can be helpful. Because there is evidence that many children with autism have diminished blood flow in certain areas of the brain and increased levels of inflammation and oxidative stress, the use of hyperbaric oxygen therapy may prove beneficial and worthwhile.

## HEART HEALTH

Hawthorn is the foundational herb for prevention and treatment of heart disease. Hawthorn dilates the arteries that supply the heart with oxygen and blood. Prolonged use of hawthorn has been shown to regulate and strengthen the heart. The standard dose can range from 500 to 1,500 milligrams a day in capsule form. Other herbs that support the cardiovascular system and reduce systemic inflammation that are easily integrated into your daily routine include garlic, green tea, turmeric, and boswellia.

Nitric oxide (NO) is an essential component of heart health and vascular function. Because NO diminishes as we age, maintaining optimal levels slows the aging process. Many plants and herbs provide natural NO; among the richest are beet greens and beet root. The Mexican herb epazote, also known as goosefoot, and the Ayurvedic herbs desmodium (*Desmodium gangeticum*) and muira puama (*Ptychopetalum olacoides*) also are beneficial. Supplements that combine beet root and hawthorn to enhance NO production are available for purchase.

## A MEAL FOR HIGH BLOOD PRESSURE

Invite your friends over for a blood pressure–lowering meal. Socializing (with human and animal friends) lowers blood pressure, as does every ingredient in the following three recipes.

### → *Carrottop Pesto* ←

Carrot greens, almonds, and garlic all lower blood pressure, so when you have a bunch of carrots and need something to do with the greens, why not make them into this delicious dinner?

**MAKES 3 TO 4 CUPS**

½ cup raw almonds

Sea salt

2 to 3 cups washed fresh carrot greens

Juice of 1 lemon

1 to 2 cloves garlic

½ cup virgin cold-pressed olive oil

Freshly ground black pepper

Lightly toast the almonds in a little olive oil, sprinkle with sea salt, and let cool thoroughly. When the almonds have cooled, add them to a food processor with the carrot greens, lemon juice, and garlic. Pulse the processor until everything is blended and then slowly add the olive oil until you are satisfied with the consistency. Add more sea salt and black pepper and serve over a baked root-vegetable mix of carrots, parsnips, potatoes, and beets.

## ⇻ *Salad with Pomegranate Dressing* ⇺

Make a large salad of grated carrots, radishes, chopped tomatoes, sliced red pepper, sliced red onion, pomegranate seeds, and slightly toasted whole pecans. Top with this pomegranate dressing.

**MAKES ABOUT ¾ CUP**

½ cup virgin cold-pressed olive oil

Juice of 1 lemon

¼ cup pomegranate juice or 1 cup fresh
    pomegranate seeds, juiced

1 garlic clove, finely chopped

1 thumb fresh ginger, grated

Make this at least an hour in advance and up to a day ahead so that the flavors blend.

Add the olive oil and lemon juice to a bowl and whisk for about half a minute. Whisk in the pomegranate juice and then add the garlic and ginger. Pour the dressing over your salad and toss just before serving. Serve at lunch or dinner with cold roselle tea (page 92).

## ⇻ *Chocolate Avocado Pudding* ⇺

This yummy, heart-healthy pudding can be prepared a day advance.

**MAKES 3 TO 4 CUPS**

1 cup coconut cream (or coconut milk)

2 ripe avocados, peeled and flesh
    removed from pit

½ cup sugar-free cocoa powder

10 to 20 drops liquid stevia or
    2 tablespoons raw dark agave

1 teaspoon glucomannan powder

⅛ cup water

½ cup toasted almond slivers

To a blender, add the coconut cream, avocado, cocoa powder, and stevia and blend until combined. In a small bowl, add the glucomannan powder and water and whisk until dissolved. Then add the mixture to the blender and blend for another 20 seconds. Pour the mixture into glass cups and place in the fridge to chill for 1 hour. Top with toasted almond slivers before serving.

## HEART PALPITATIONS

Heart palpitations are a common symptom during menopause. Strengthen adrenal function with adaptogens and reduce caffeine, which can be a trigger.

The powdered seeds of Chinese jujube (*Ziziphus jujuba*) have been shown to reduce palpitations, and they are also a potent anxiolytic and sleep aid. The powder combines well with the seeds or powder of griffonia (*Griffonia simplicifolia*). You can eat the fresh or dried fruits, take an extract, or add the powder to your daily healthy heart smoothie (recipe follows).

> ⟫   *Healthy Heart Smoothie*   ⟪

Create a daily smoothie with the herbs and foods listed here, adding berries as a rich source of antioxidants. You can vary the ingredients as needed for specific symptoms and to keep the smoothie interesting over time. Cocoa is rich in polyphenols, which support endothelial function and reduce inflammation, thus reducing risk of stroke or heart attack. The endothelium is a thin membrane that lines the heart and blood vessels and is responsible for relaxing the blood vessels and ensuring adequate blood flow. Diabetes and hypertension can harm endothelium function. The amino acid taurine can be dosed up to 1,000 milligrams a day to reduce hypertension. (Hypotension is less common, but thiamine can be used to increase blood pressure.) After age sixty, hematocrit levels rise in women, whereas during menses the monthly loss of blood keeps hematocrit sufficiently low, offering heart protection. Hematocrit is the ratio of the volume of red blood cells to the total volume of blood. It can be artificially high due to dehydration, but if you are adequately hydrated and it remains high, you may need to reduce hematocrit levels as an added protective factor. Dr. Jonathan Wright recommends that women donate blood as often as necessary to maintain premenopause hematocrit levels of 42 in order to reduce the risk of heart attack and stroke. If you are concerned about your risk of cardiovascular disease, obtain a blood viscosity test, which measures the thickness and stickiness of your blood and the ease at which it flows through the arteries. If blood viscosity is high, then you can add 250 milligrams of nattokinase powder to this smoothie as an anticoagulant. Nattokinase offers a safe alternative to low-dose aspirin use, which causes increased risk of bleeding and death.

**CAUTION:** Check with with your prescriber about using nattokinase if you are already on a blood thinner.

**MAKES 1 SERVING**

½ cup unsweetened pomegranate juice

½ tablespoon matcha tea

1 cup blueberries

1 plum, stone removed

1 teaspoon hawthorn berry powder

½ teaspoon ground turmeric or
    1 teaspoon fresh turmeric juice

½ teaspoon ground boswellia

1 thumb fresh ginger or 1 teaspoon fresh
    ginger juice

**OPTIONAL HERBAL ADDITIONS**

1 teaspoon ground jujube (for heart
    palpitations)

200 milligrams griffonia (for heart
    palpitations and anxiety)

Ground cayenne pepper (to enhance
    circulation)

500 to 1,000 milligrams taurine (for
    high blood pressure)

Add all the ingredients to a blender and blend until combined. This smoothie can serve as your foundational smoothie to drink daily. Add any of the optional herbs to target your individual needs.

## ATRIAL FIBRILLATION

Atrial fibrillation, or A-fib, emotional stress, and heart rhythm are all connected. In A-fib, the heart's two upper chambers beat chaotically and do not coordinate with the two lower chambers of the heart. A-fib increases during periods of mourning, especially the death of a partner, and there is an increased risk of heart attack during the first twenty-four hours of bereavement. This acute stress creates increased levels of stress hormones, which make blood "stickier" and more likely to clot. The protocol for managing A-fib, whether it is due to grief or another process, involves enhancing overall heart function and thinning the blood naturally with the following protocol. In addition to this A-fib herbal protocol, the Heart Math Freeze-Frame and Heart Lock-In methods are attitudinal and meditation methods that help to reregulate heart rhythms, are pleasant and fun to do, and can be learned at home via online training.

⇻ *A-Fib Protocol* ⇺

This protocol can be done daily for as long as necessary.

- 500 milligrams hawthorn extract, 3 times a day
- 100 milligrams nattokinase (a fermented product from soy), 2 times a day

- 2 to 4 grams fish oil once a day
- 200 milligrams CoQ10 once a day

### THE MYTH OF HIGH CHOLESTEROL

The danger of high cholesterol is one of the biggest health myths out there, and it goes hand in hand with the myth that eating eggs or healthy fat is bad for your cholesterol. In fact, cholesterol that is too low is more dangerous than cholesterol that is too high. Cholesterol is needed for brain health, and low cholesterol is a risk factor for anxiety.

Berberine-rich herbs or supplements can be used to lower cholesterol if it is worrisome, but lowering inflammation and supporting your arteries are more important to heart health and both can be done with hawthorn. Chocolate is an excellent food for cholesterol balance and vascular health. Statins are dangerous medications and should be avoided. Dr. Beatrice Golomb has conducted extensive research on the dangers of statins to women's health. She has found that they can cause memory loss, neurological diseases, and rhabdomyolysis, a condition that leads to the death of muscle fibers and kidney disease.

# COGNITIVE PERFORMANCE, DEMENTIA, AND ALZHEIMER'S DISEASE

A healthy heart often means a healthy mind, and poor heart health often leads to cognitive decline and dementia. We can also experience mild cognitive decline as we age. When we consider supporting our cognitive function, whether we want to be more productive and focused, sharpen our memory, or slow the aging of the brain, we can use a combination of herbs to support the interrelated functions of increased blood flow and lower inflammation, lubricate neuronal communication with fats, enrich the neurotransmitters, reduce cortisol, and manage glucose.

There are many wonderful herbal medicines to use for improving our cognitive function. The herbs that support our focus and performance in our early years are the same ones we use, perhaps at higher doses, as we age. Herbal medicines and healthy foods, supplemented with amino acids and nutrients, will prevent and treat many symptoms of impaired cognition and enable the reduction or total elimination of pharmaceutical medications. It is safer for the brain to use herbs and nutrition rather than medications to enhance focus, attention, and memory.

## PERFORMANCE AND MEMORY COCKTAIL

Plants that especially enhance blood flow to the brain include ginkgo and vinpocetine, a compound derived from the lesser periwinkle plant (*Vinca minor*). Nervines and adaptogens like ashwagandha support memory, reduce stress, and lower blood glucose. Fats from the seeds of evening primrose, borage, hemp, and flax lube the neuronal connections in the brain. Whole eggs enhance acetylcholine, the memory chemical in the brain. Nutritional support should include the mineral lithium orotate (20 to 40 milligrams a day) and phosphatidylserine (200 milligrams a day).

### → *Daily Snacks for Cognitive Health* ←

- ½ cup lycium berries (i.e., goji berries or wolfberries)
- 1 cup blueberries
- 10 raw almonds
- ½ cup raw pumpkin seeds
- ½ cup sardines or canned wild Alaskan salmon
- 1 to 2 eggs
- 1 cup raw broccoli dipped in flaxseed and olive oil aioli
- 1 to 2 espresso shots

### → *Midmorning Haritaki Memory Tea* ←

**MAKES 1 SERVING**

Haritaki (*Terminalia chebula*) is called the King of Medicines in Tibet and is one of the all-important triphala compounds of Ayurveda. The Medicine Buddha is often depicted holding the fruit, which enhances acute memory, energy, and focus, so drink this tea early in the day. Make haritaki tea like you would cowgirl coffee. Add 2 tablespoons of haritaki powder to 2 cups of boiling water, simmer for 2 minutes, strain, and drink.

> ↠  *Midday Sage Memory Tea*  ↞

**MAKES 1 SERVING**

Spanish sage (*Salvia officinalis*), garden sage (*Salvia officinalis*), and red sage (*Salvia miltiorrhiza*) all make memory teas and can be used individually or combined. Add 1 ounce of fresh leaves or ½ ounce of dried leaves to 2 cups of boiling water. Let infuse for 30 to 60 minutes, strain, and drink 1 to 2 cups per day.

**CAUTION:** This tea has a mild laxative effect and should not be used during pregnancy or nursing.

> ↠  *Bioidentical Hormones: Memory, Heart, and Bones*  ↞

Bioidentical hormones are essential, starting in perimenopause and increasing through menopause. The science is clear that maintaining hormone levels supports women's cognitive memory, heart, and bone health. This is one area that herbs play a supporting role, but they cannot do it all alone. Hormones to consider with your prescriber include melatonin, estrogen, DHEA, testosterone, and progesterone, all of which contribute protection to cognitive function.

## THE ApoE GENE AND UNDERSTANDING YOUR RISK FOR ALZHEIMER'S DISEASE

Mild cognitive decline used to be considered part of normal aging, but it is now recognized as a precursor to dementia or Alzheimer's. Women have a higher risk of developing dementia and Alzheimer's than do men.

Alzheimer's is one type of dementia that has a genetic risk factor based on our ApoE gene status. The ApoE gene controls the production of the protein apolipoprotein E, which mixes with fats to form molecules called lipoproteins. Lipoproteins are responsible for transporting cholesterol through the bloodstream. The ApoE gene has three alleles, or alternate forms: ε2, ε3, and ε4. The ε3 allele is the most common and is found in more than 50 percent of the general population. The ε4 allele is the largest risk factor for late-life onset of Alzheimer's disease. Having one ε4 allele increases the risk factor of getting Alzheimer's by 30 percent. Two alleles of ε4 increase the risk to 70 percent or more, and 40 to 65 percent of people with Alzheimer's have at least one copy of the ε4 allele.

However, having one or two ε4s is not all bad news! While it was previously thought that Alzheimer's was not preventable or modifiable, there are many factors that can reduce risk, including intensive plant-based and herbal nutrition rich in anti-inflammatories and adaptogens, low saturated fats, a low glycemic diet, exercise, detoxification, and the following herbal supports I discuss. In essence the philosophy and methods I describe throughout this book all support a healthy brain.

## → Test: What Is My ApoE Status? ←

To find out your genetic risk you can take a simple salivary gene test for your ApoE status. Knowledge is power. It is advisable to maintain confidentiality about the test results and even consider using a pseudonym as it is unknown if and how results may be used by insurance companies or long-term care organizations. (See "Resources.")

## → Daily Dementia Prevention Protocol ←

Make a daily prevention smoothie and supplement with herbal compounds in capsules and teas. You may mix and combine herbal powders or extracts to achieve the blend and taste you like. This combination enhances brain function and cognition.

**MAKES 2 SERVINGS**

1½ cups hemp or almond milk

¾ cup blueberries

½ cup unsweetened pomegranate juice

300 to 500 micrograms huperzine
   (an extract of Chinese club moss)

½ teaspoon green tea powder

50 milligrams rhodiola extract

60 milligrams vinpocetine extract

300 milligrams bacopa extract (with total
   bacoside content of 55 percent of
   extract)

2,000 milligrams gotu kola powder

750 milligrams curcumin powder

30 milligrams piperine or ½ teaspoon
   black pepper

1 thumb ginger or ½ teaspoon fresh
   ginger juice

300 milligrams St. John's wort

200 milligrams magnolia bark extract

100 milligrams yuan zhi powdered
   extract

1,000 milligrams lion's mane mushroom

500 milligrams brain glandular powder

1,000 milligrams citicoline powder

½ teaspoon hemp seed oil

½ teaspoon chia seeds (optional, if
   constipated)

Add all the ingredients to a blender and blend until combined. This smoothie can be made and adjusted to body weight and age and divided into 2 doses, one taken in the morning and one in the midafternoon.

## TREATMENT COCKTAIL: MIDDLE- TO LATE-STAGE ALZHEIMER'S AND DEMENTIA

Mid- to late-stage Alzheimer's and dementia treatment focuses on slowing the degenerative process and managing anxiety and circadian rhythm disruption that leads to sundowning, a state of late-afternoon agitation. At this stage swallowing pills can be difficult, and sipping a smoothie is a lot easier.

### → *Smoothie for Agitation and Anxiety* ←

**MAKES 1 SERVING**

¾ cup oat or hemp milk

1 cup frozen blueberries

½ teaspoon green tea powder

30 milligrams vinpocetine

300 milligrams St. John's wort

1 teaspoon hemp oil

Raw local honey or stevia to taste

Add all the ingredients to a blender and blend until combined. Drink once or twice a day.

**OPTIONS:** To further reduce anxiety during the daytime add either 200 to 400 milligrams (60 milligrams kavalactones) of kava or 400 to 1,200 milligrams of valerian, hops, and passionflower to the smoothie.

To improve sleep during the night, add 600 milligrams of sage or 1,200 milligrams of valerian, hops, and passionflower at bedtime and remove the green tea from this blend as it can be stimulating.

### → *Other Remedies for Reducing Anxiety Before Bedtime* ←

- 3 milligrams melatonin liposomal spray
- 1 cup chamomile tea
- Exposure to full spectrum light
- Lemon balm aromatherapy, in a diffuser or massage oil

# WEIGHT LOSS, WEIGHT GAIN, AND BODY CONDITIONING

I weighed over 10 pounds when I was born, and the doctors and nurses joked to my parents that I could get up and walk home right then and there. By age twelve, at 145 pounds, I was a competitive athlete and my weight (and lean body mass) kept going up and up. The gifts of my genetics derive from my ancestors who pushed oxen in the fields of Eastern Europe for eight hours day. When I spent six hours a day on a tennis court, I came close to that, and that's what my body needs; however, it's not what my body gets in my sixth decade. So, I focus on body conditioning—modern life's equivalent to pushing oxen—lifting weights, daily intensive interval training, yoga, and balance.

In spite of all the civil rights movements of the past 100 years, the any-size-and-body-is-beautiful movement has been slow to gain traction. As we explore herbal medicine and weight loss, I want to shift our focus from body size and its myriad values in modern society to understanding muscle and fat, and how herbs help build strong bodies. We actually weigh more when we have more muscle, and muscle is our engine, stamina, strength, and balance. Converting fat to muscle is our goal, not weight loss, per se. Muscle helps regulate glucose uptake, and it helps keep us pain free. While the following section explores some herbs that help weight loss, these herbs work best to increase muscle, enhance glucose uptake, balance hormones, eliminate fluid retention, and enhance overall metabolism.

The keys to body conditioning (which may include the side effect of weight loss) are as follows:

- Identifying how you feel, not how others make you feel

- Building muscle

- Raising the heart rate consistently through interval training

- Getting 8 to 9 hours of sleep a night

- Eliminating grains and most of the "white" foods

- Reducing cortisol levels by reducing stress

- Reducing systemic inflammation

- Lowering blood sugar

- Eating healthy proteins and fats

- Eating plenty of plant fiber to enhance satiety

- Being sure you don't go hungry

- Refraining from dieting

The principles of being in condition and feeling good about our bodies include using herbs that enhance satiety, decrease inflammation, decrease blood glucose and enhance insulin uptake, increase metabolism, and reduce stress.

## WEIGHT LOSS

Weight, like many health concerns, is a complex mix of epigenetics, which is the study of how environmental exposures like food and sedentariness activate (or don't activate) our genetic responses. This includes the science of our body's fat/lean mass ratio and here, there's very little "give." Research consistently identifies a "set point," the weight at which the body seems to want to return and stay, regardless of interventions. Even bariatric surgery is no guarantee of maintaining weight loss, and it brings with it a high risk of malnutrition, depression, alcoholism, and suicidality. Nevertheless, herbs enhance many of our efforts to shape the body we want.

Here, I explore some principles of weight loss, fat loss, and muscle gain that focus on herbal medicines. Remember, don't do all of these interventions at once. Be gentle with your body and choose only one or two herbs or smoothies for a 3-month period to judge results.

### TRIPHALA AYURVEDA

Triphala is a traditional Ayurvedic formula that contains three fruits native to India, amla, bibhitaki (*Terminalia belerica*), and haritaki. Triphala helps cleanse and nourish the whole body, with a focus on the digestive system. The three fruits work synergistically to support healthy respiratory, urinary, cardiovascular, reproductive, and urinary systems. Because it facilitates digestion and elimination, triphala is suggested as a part of a weight-loss regimen. If you get diarrhea, you are taking too much. The best time to take triphala is on an empty stomach upon waking or right before bed. An Ayurvedic principle is to fully taste herbs we take, so even if you don't love the taste of these herbs, it's worth trying it first as a tea. It can also be taken as a powder, extract, or capsule (1,000 to 2,000 milligrams a day).

**CARALLUMA FIMBRIATA (*Caralluma adscendens* var. *fimbriata*)**

An edible cactus rich in nutrients and fiber that reduces food cravings, caralluma fimbriata is available in a standardized extract called slimaluma. Standard dose is 500 milligrams twice a day.

**NOPALE CACTUS (*Opuntia ficus-indica*)**

This readily available edible cactus can be found in many large grocery stores and especially in Mexican groceries. It lowers blood glucose and increases satiety. It is an ideal food for hypoglycemia and diabetes. Fresh nopales can also be cooked and mixed with eggs and ground cayenne pepper, which increases satiety and reduces sensations of hunger. Nopale is also available as a powder and can be added to smoothies. A nopale smoothie is delicious, satisfying, and soothing to digestion (see Nopale and Roselle Fat Loss Smoothie below).

**ANTI-INFLAMMATORY HERBS FOR WEIGHT BALANCE**

Excess fat in the body releases inflammatory cytokines and reduces the capacity of the body to use glucose efficiently. Reducing inflammation has a bidirectional effect: it helps to reduce obesity and sets the stage for building muscle. Exercise can increase short-term inflammatory response, which results in muscle building, so a daily anti-inflammatory herb will be important to your overall regimen.

**Roselle**

I love roselle and write about it extensively in chapter 4 (see page 91), where you will also find some recipes. It is one of the most inexpensive anti-inflammatory herbs. Roselle supports healthy weight loss, lowers blood pressure, and enhances glucose uptake in the body. Drink 1 cup of tea (page 92) every day for as long as you desire.

---

### ⇅ *Nopale and Roselle Fat Loss Smoothie* ⇇

**MAKES 1 SERVING**

1 cup strong roselle tea

1 cup fresh-cut nopale cactus

1 teaspoon chia seeds

¼ fresh avocado or 1 teaspoon coconut oil

10 drops stevia

Add all the ingredients to a blender and blend until combined. Drink for lunch or as a snack daily for as long as you like.

---

## HERBS THAT ENHANCE METABOLISM AND INSULIN SENSITIVITY

A member of the gourd family, jiaogulan (*Gynostemma pentaphyllum*) is called the Herb of Immortality as it is used like other adaptogens. It is an antioxidant that lowers cholesterol and has been studied for its ability to switch on kinase, or AMPK, the "master metabolic regulator," leading to a reduction in fat and improved insulin resistance. It is energizing and should be used only in the morning and early afternoon. Start off with the lowest dose and note your response and results. Make 2 to 4 cups of tea daily or take capsules containing an extract of 75 milligrams of 30 percent gypenosides, 1 to 3 times a day.

CAUTION: It may stimulate immune function and should be avoided in people with autoimmune disorders. It is also a mild blood thinner. Too much intake may lead to diarrhea.

African mango (*Irvingia gabonensis*) supports leptin and insulin sensitivity, which is often diminished in long-term overweight individuals. Take 150 milligrams twice a day and rotate its use with other herbs every 3 months.

## FAT LOSS AND THERMOGENICS

There are several herbs and constituents, notably caffeine, that increase body heat and metabolism. These thermogenic herbs increase the body's metabolic rate; they "heat" things up. However, their use should just be a part of your overall protocol since too much caffeine can backfire and increase cortisol, leading to fat increase and strain on the heart.

### Barberry/Berberine

Berberine, an extract from barberry, helps blood glucose levels and has been shown to reduce blood lipid levels, resulting in weight loss. Take 500 milligrams 3 times a day for 3 months and then rotate to use of other herbs.

### Green Tea/Matcha Tea

Matcha tea has been shown to help burn fat. You can easily make it part of your diet by adding the powder or a strong matcha infusion to a smoothie like the following.

## → Thermo-Mocha Smoothie ←

**MAKES 1 SERVING**

1 cup hemp or almond milk

½ heaping teaspoon matcha green tea powder (or substitute 1 cup strong matcha tea and reduce milk by half)

1 tablespoon cocoa

⅓ cup coffee

Pinch of ground cayenne pepper

⅛ teaspoon ground cardamom

10 drops stevia

One to two 500 milligram capsules berberine (optional)

Add all of the ingredients to a blender and blend until combined. Drink as a morning drink, daily as desired.

---

### DIURETIC HERBS FOR FLUID RETENTION AND EDEMA

Carrying extra fluid can make us feel bloated and heavy. The causes of fluid retention include eating grains and flour products, high blood pressure, and, paradoxically, dehydration. Increasing foods rich in magnesium and potassium (and reducing sodium-rich foods for a short time) can be helpful.

Tamarind (see Agua de Tamarindo on page 129) is a gentle diuretic and mild laxative. Drink daily for 7 days. Celery and parsley are also diuretic plants that can be juiced fresh as "mini shots" once a day for up to 10 days at a time. Then take a break for 10 days.

Skin brushing has many benefits, including stimulating the lymphatic system and releasing fluids.

## WEIGHT GAIN

The principal for weight gain is the same as weight loss: ensure an adequate level of muscle and fat, but don't worry about weight per se. Increasing muscle mass improves strength and energy. Some people gain weight with a complex carbohydrate–rich diet and others with mostly protein and fat. Knowing your metabolism and what gives you more energy will illuminate the right mix of fuel for you. Good-quality fats are essential and a mix of olive oil, sesame oil, raw butter (even leaf lard), and evening primrose are important for hormonal health.

## → *Weight-Gain Smoothie* ←

**MAKES 1 SERVING**

2 tablespoons whey protein isolate

1 cup whole fat Greek yogurt

1 tablespoon collagen powder

1 frozen banana

½ cup favorite berries (or 1 heaping
tablespoon cocoa with a few pinches
of sea salt)

2 tablespoons almond or cashew butter

½ teaspoon evening primrose oil

½ tablespoon raw local honey

Add all of the ingredients to a blender and blend until combined. Drink once a day.

# HERBAL SUPPORT AT THE END OF LIFE

The process of dying may last days or weeks, and people may be confined to a chair or bed; they may be anxious, in pain, or at peace. We never know in advance. I have had friends who were anxious all their lives and became very peaceful at this time, and I have had friends who meditated for decades preparing for a calm transition and who, not long before death, suffered from brain damage that made them act aggressively. I have worked with some people who, before they take to bed, have a spiritual anxiety about the future and what happens after death, and for this there are several supports, including the use of the psilocybin mushroom under the supervision of a specialist.

At this time our focus is on support care, pain relief, connection when it is desired, and quietude when it is requested. It is a gift to be able to be part of someone's leave-taking, though often not simple or easy. Some people enter a nonverbal state but are very much aware of visitors and benefit from physical and nonverbal touch and comfort. Some senses, usually touch and smell, remain strong, and others like sight and hearing may fade. I have had a number of opportunities to facilitate gentle foot or hand massages or rocking, using aromas that are comforting and anxiety reducing, and often there is little to do but be present. One need not know any special massage method; just follow intuition and be gentle. At this stage it is about light, soothing touch with very little pressure, and the aromas will have a positive effect. If people are responsive, you can ask them if they want their hands or feet touched and give them an option of a few aromas. If they are nonresponsive, you can start with the feet and choose an aroma. If the individual does not want to be touched, they may still enjoy the aroma, in which case you can place a diffuser in the room or just rub a few drops of oil on your hands and place your hands near their nostrils for a few moments. If you know your loved one's favorite aroma, use that, but if you don't, choose from the following essential oils.

ESSENTIAL OILS FOR END OF LIFE CARE

- **Pain reduction**—Chamomile aromatherapy and foot and hand massage

- **End of life nausea or digestive upset**—Vanilla can be applied in a diffuser or added to an almond massage oil

- **Anxiety and restlessness**—Lavender or helichrysum (*Helichrysum italicum*) aromatherapy

- **Increased energy and focus for conversation**—Either peppermint and citrus oils can be used with a diffuser. Open an orange and allow your loved one to enjoy the fresh aroma or places some drops of juice on her lips (use separately).

- **Calm and peace**—Palo santo (*Bursera graveolens*) in a diffuser

- **Hiccups or intestinal pain**—Rose oil rubbed on the inner wrist, the tip of the breastbone, and where the vagus nerve comes to the surface on the ear lobe.

## HICCUPS

Hiccups are a common, often serious problem during the late stages of dying. They are spasms of the diaphragm and irritation of the vagus and/or phrenic nerves and can result for a number of reasons. Hiccups can last up to forty-eight hours, two to thirty days, or longer than thirty days. Conventionally, antipsychotic convulsion medications are given, but try the following protocol first.

→ *Hiccups Protocol* ←

- Provide an antispasmodic tincture containing black cohosh root, myrrh resin, skullcap flowering tops, skunk cabbage root, lobelia, and cayenne pepper. (See the "Antispasmodic" section on pages 34–35.)

- Follow this an hour later with the Ayurvedic remedy of ½ teaspoon of cardamom powder simmered in 1 cup of water until reduced to half a cup. Drink warm.

- Both THC and CBD are anticonvulsants and can be used as a tincture, oil, or vapor to stop hiccups.

## BODYWORK TECHNIQUES FOR HICCUPS

If this protocol does not help, there are a couple of other bodywork methods that you can try. One is to apply gentle pressure and massage to the hard palate inside the "roof" of the mouth. The other is to gently massage the earlobe (it's a vagus nerve contact).

## RECTAL MASSAGE TECHNIQUE

This technique can be used for chronic hiccups lasting more than a few hours. I have used it with success with an individual who had hiccups for twelve days, round the clock. The client was unresponsive to every other intervention. Prolonged hiccups that last for several or more days can occur because of gastric distress or after respiratory distress, such as pneumonia, when the phrenic nerve is irritated. Hiccups are also common during the dying process.

Begin with "Perineal Antispasmodic Relaxation Technique" phases 1 and 2 (see page 35). Once you've completed these two phases, initiate phase 3. Ask the individual to lie on whatever side is most comfortable and place one pillow between the legs and another under the head. Sitting behind the patient, use your thumb and forefinger to apply gentle pressure to the earlobe from front to back; this will contact the vagus nerve. With the other hand, gently insert a gloved, well-lubricated little finger just inside the rectum and gently and very slowly apply very light pressure around the anal sphincter, which will also relax the vagus nerve. Hold this position for up to 20 minutes for the treatment to take effect.

## SUPPORTING CAREGIVERS

So many of us are caregivers, providing care for ill individuals of any age at some point in our lives. I was fortunate to be able to care for my mother who had Alzheimer's. I felt it was a deep service to facilitate the challenges my mother faced as her mind and body stopped working over the decade as she neared death. I also had to work diligently to take care of myself while I had my own family and full-time work, and I certainly felt the stress. I was fortunate to engage other caregivers to support me as I could not do it alone. I found a geriatric care manager who was able to advise me so I had an independent perspective on all the care options, and the local Area Agency on Aging, found in every community in the United States, provided immeasurable support.

Emotional and biological stress paves the way for caregiver illness. Caregiving is a marathon, and it includes the ups and downs of diagnoses, doctor's appointments, decisions, and treatment challenges. Especially since as dementia progresses, so does the patient's agitation and distress, which only adds to our own.

The herbs that are most important at this time are the adaptogens for resilience, hypoglycemic herbs to stabilize blood glucose, immunomodulators to stay healthy, and sedatives for deep rest at night. This smoothie also makes a quick meal on the run that will sustain you for several hours.

### ↠ *Caregiver Resilience Smoothie* ↞

Make enough café de capomo in advance and keep it in the fridge so you can use it daily. A substitute for capomo is a shot of coffee, but remember—too much coffee will exhaust, where a small amount provides a boost.

**MAKES 1 SERVING**

½ cup hemp milk

½ cup Café de Capomo (page 61)

½ teaspoon ashwagandha

½ teaspoon maca

1 teaspoon bee pollen

1 to 2 capsules powdered free
   amino acids

1 tablespoon tahini or almond butter

5 drops liquid stevia

Add the ingredients to the blender and blend until smooth. You can also add 2 to 3 ice cubes if you like. Drink daily.

## CONCLUSION

I have learned much about healing with herbs as a result of my own wounding, and I embrace the idea of the "wounded healer" as one of the most useful ways to deal with adversities or challenges that occur in our lives. Most cultures and religions tell stories about the ways in which illness or wounding occurs, quickens personal growth, and then initiates the process of becoming the hero and the healer. This is not to suggest that we seek out our wounding or that we "ask for it" or that our mental attitude invited the adverse experience, as some popular discourse suggests. Wounding is a universal experience, and while it can lead to transmutation of one's trauma, it also often leaves us with scars, pain, and an altered life. One needs no illness or trauma to grow; it's just that there is little else to do with traumatic experiences except transform them for our own benefit, and perhaps for the benefit of others.

Herbs are our allies in this transformation; they help us heal from illnesses, and they smooth out the bumps in our life cycles. They are always most generous when they reveal that, like each branch, root, leaf, and bud they share, we are also part of nature and have our seat in the cosmos.

## ⇻ 8 ⇺

# HERBAL RITUALS

Rituals are organized ceremonies conducted individually or with other people that focus our intention, synchronize our rhythms, and deepen our connection to ourselves, to others, and to the cosmos. While "rituals" are usually associated with a practice or pattern of behavior regularly performed in a set manner—such as family seating arrangements around the dinner table—the term has a deeper meaning when applied to a more venerable practice. While many of us grew up practicing rituals, often associated with religious or spiritual practices, they may have sometimes felt empty, or we may not have felt connected to the process or the symbols used. Rituals are meant to help us align with our deepest self, our community, and the unseen world. When a ritual is successful, we feel fulfilled and satisfied.

The ingredients of a successful ritual (whether it is just for you, a small group of close friends, or even a large gathering) are that you imbue it with meaning, symbols, and sensory experiences that are important to you. Herbs, incense, music, and other objects allow us to concentrate our focus and energy into a desired outcome. They provide an opportunity to align our energy with the other participants while we share something to drink and eat and to seal one's personal and group internal experiences.

## USING INCENSE IN RITUALS AND CEREMONIES

The use of incense can be an important contribution to healing and spiritual rituals. Incense is burned to create a fragrance in order to affect our mood, cleanse a space, and encourage spiritual connection and group cohesion. Incense is most often made from a gum or resin derived from many of the herbs whose flowers, bark, and leaves we use as medicine internally or topically. Incense should be used sparingly, briefly, and for ritual and ceremonial purposes. Like all plant medicines, the quality of the incense is important. As you read through these different types of incense, choose the ones that appeal to you and sample their aromas. It is also worth considering how they are used traditionally so you might incorporate these elements into the rituals that follow.

CAUTION: The burning of incense indoors should be considered for any potential toxicity or irritation, especially if members of the household have asthma or respiratory conditions.

## CEDAR

The cedar tree is central to the lives and health of native peoples of the Northwest Coast of North America. Traditional longhouses are made of cedar, and burning cedar is an integral part of many native ceremonies as it is renowned for its healing and spiritual powers. The wood and leaves have antifungal, antibacterial, and insecticidal properties. The Kwakiutl and Coast Salish people use cedarwood with afterbirth to ensure a long healthy life of a newborn. The Kwakiutl wrap the afterbirth in the four layers of cedar bark and bury it in a place where it will be walked over, such as a threshold. The Coast Salish people place the afterbirth in an old, healthy cedarwood stump. Shaved cedarwood is used as a vulnerary and bandage, and yellow cedar (*Cupressus nootkatensis*) is used in sweat baths to help one regain strength after illness.

## COPAL

Copal is the name of a resin from various trees called copal, including most commonly *Protium copal, Bursera bipinnata, Pinus pseudostrobus*, and *Bursera graveolens*, which are native to Mexico and Central America. It was most commonly used in southern Mexico among the Maya and the Mazatec during mushroom ceremonies to accompany trance states. Copal incense is available in small disks, small pieces, or on a stick and has a sweet smoky smell.

Traditionally, copal, which is also referred to as the "blood of trees," is paired with maize (corn) and used in offerings to the gods. It is also very common to bury the dead under or near the copal tree. Prior to contact with Europeans, Nahua women in Mexico held esteemed positions where they chose the copal tree for burial rites.

### FRANKINCENSE (*Boswellia sacra*)

Frankincense is resin from the genus *Boswellia*, of which there are four species. Frankincense was used by pre-Abrahamic religions and then later integrated into Judaism and Christianity as a consecrated aroma. It was one of the gifts given to baby Jesus by the biblical Magi. It is also one of the oldest commodities known to have been traded by the ancient Egyptians, who bought the resin (along with myrrh) from the Phoenicians to be used as an insect repellent, perfume, incense, healing ointment, and embalming ointment. It is used in Ayurvedic medicine as a purification aroma. The two active constituents in boswellia are boswellin and boswellic acid, which are known to be anti-inflammatory and antiarthritic. Boswellia taken internally is used for arthritis and colitis. The Jewish Yemenite women use boswellia as an aid to childbirth by burning the resin and letting the smoke rise up into the vaginal cavity, allowing for a less painful delivery.

### MYRRH

The fragrant resin from the *Commiphora* genus is often used in conjunction with frankincense. Its religious and spiritual influence dates back to ancient Egypt. Myrrh is an essential part of childbirth in Somalia, where it is called *qataf* and is burned in the house of a woman who has just given birth and given to newborns in a diluted mixture.

Myrrh is also used as a topical analgesic and oral antiseptic, acting on the opiate receptors in the brain. In Chinese Medicine, myrrh is regarded as a "blood mover" and is prescribed for circulatory and uterine-related complications.

### PALO SANTO

Common in Mexico and Central and South America, palo santo (or sacred or holy stick) is used for its purifying properties and for calming the mind. It is also among many woods that are referred to as "copal." Its aromatic wood and oil can be burned, or the oil can be added to diffusers.

### SANDALWOOD

Sandalwood oil is harvested from the wood of trees in the genus *Santalum*. Its popularity threatens the trees' extinction, especially because they are slow-growing trees. The use of sandalwood in rituals and in temples and places of worship is an ancient practice of many of the world's religions. The ancient Egyptians used sandalwood for embalming the dead and in the worship of their deities, the Buddhists burn sandalwood along with cloves, the Zoroastrians use the wood in the ever-burning fire in their temples, and Hindu Ayurvedic practitioners prepare a paste from the wood to use in rituals and ceremonies. Burning sandalwood enhances relaxation and the practice of meditation.

### SWEETGRASS

Sweetgrass (*Hierochloe odorata*) is a plant sacred to many indigenous peoples in North America and is used in prayer, cleansing ceremonies, and offerings and for purification. The Anishinabe, Bode'wad mi, and Odawa people consider sweetgrass, along with tobacco, cedar, and sage, to be one of the four most important medicines for healing. Blackfeet tribal women drink the tea to stop bleeding after childbirth and to help expel afterbirth. Referred to as the "hair of mother earth," the grass has a sweet smell that comes from coumarin, a natural anticoagulant, which is also found in cinnamon, sweet clover, and cherry blossoms.

### WHITE SAGE

The burning of white sage has long been used in the practice called "smudging," where the sage smoke is fanned over a body or around a person. It is commonly used among indigenous Americans for purification and cleansing rituals. The Cahuilla and the Kumeyaay peoples use sage as a febrifuge and pulmonary aid in sweat lodges. Burning sage is a powerful antiseptic and air disinfectant and has been shown to be helpful for pulmonary, neurological, and dermatological conditions.

## CREATING A RITUAL FOR EACH LIFE STAGE

When I create rituals, I often call upon the energies of Freya, the pre-Christian Norse *volva*, or shaman. She is the one who sees the future and creates reality through her ritual magic based on the strength of her intention and attention. Freya also enjoys her pleasures, so rituals that call upon Freya might include some sweets, such as wine, honey, and cake. I have organized these rituals in groups according to a progression that provides us with an opportunity and structure to recognize, honor, and celebrate our many stages of life. The following rituals are jumping off points for your own creativity and meaning making.

## CREATING YOUR HERBAL LOVE AID KIT AND ALTAR

When I was thirty-five, I had a painful breakup of a long-term relationship. I knew in my heart that I would one day in the future meet someone new but that I needed time to heal and grow. The time came five years later when I told my friends that I felt that I was ready to meet a new life companion. My friend Brooke gave me a dime-store diamond ring that had been passed on to her and that she had used in her own love ritual. She suggested that I make an altar and put this on it. I also chose myrrh incense to burn, and then I wrote a list of the twenty attributes I was seeking in my partner-to-be.

It was fun and meaningful to create my altar, but the part about it that was most powerful was to sit down and actually define who it was that I wanted to have join me on my life path. What did I have to offer someone? What did I want someone to offer me? So I made a list with three columns: (1) requirements, (2) nice attributes to have but not essential, and (3) deal breakers. I thus created my altar, adding the ring, three bowls of water, peony flowers, and myrrh, and I made a commitment to sit at it every day for a few minutes, breathing and contemplating on the nature of love. The bowls of water represented the flow of life and also my lack of attachment to the outcome. On the one hand I was placing my intention and focus on the outcome, and on the other I was allowing for no outcome. This is an ideal frame of mind. I burned myrrh incense because engaging self-love is an important requisite for finding the love of another. Once I had finished my "list of twenty," I added it to the altar, placing it under a small beeswax votive candle that I burned each time I sat. I left the altar in place, and I put it all aside in my mind.

During this time, I had also been thinking for a while of going back for my doctorate, and a few months after making my altar I signed up for graduate school. The first entry conference was in New York in August, but at the last moment I had to cancel that start date because of work. I then signed up to begin three months later in November, in Washington, D.C., but the night before I was to begin I had to cancel because of a wave of uncharacteristic and overwhelming panic. I couldn't figure it out, so I decided to honor it and cancel my start date again. I then decided to sign up to begin, now, two months later in January, in San Diego, and this time I kept the date.

Upon arrival I entered the conference room to start my class, and a man walked up to me and was very engaging. As a somewhat reserved Bostonian, I thought, "Whoa, he is much too friendly," and I ignored him. He came up to me again at the break and again I thought, "What does this buster want anyway?" The next day he approached me again, and again and again over the ensuing days, and each time I gave him a gentle brush-off. Then one day he came up to me and this time I paid attention to him, and truly for the first time looked into his eyes and realized that this man was someone with whom I should talk. We began by talking about our studies and our writing and work lives, and it was clear we had a lot to share and we were simpatico. Near the end of the ten-day conference, he shared with me about how he had decided to go to graduate school at this middle-aged time in his life. He told me that he had first planned to start in New York in August, but then had to cancel due to work. And then he had rescheduled for Washington, D.C., in November, but again at the last minute, work caused a delay. So then he settled on starting at this moment in San Diego—all just exactly as I had done. This is how I met my future husband, who by the way, turned out to have all the attributes (and none of the deal breakers) on my "list of twenty," which was still sitting on my altar.

You can create a love altar that means something to you using dime-store rings, herbs, flowers, candles, rocks, and incense, along with your all-important "list of 20." But remember, when your loved one appears before you, you must open your eyes and recognize that what you have been asking for has indeed arrived!

## PRE-WEDDING/COMMITMENT CEREMONY RITUAL

During this ritual gathering, the bride's female friends and family gather to support the bride in celebrating her next steps by relinquishing the past, including regrets, that may get in her way.

Rue is the herb used in this ritual. It offers protection and cleansing, but traditionally it is associated with regrets; hence the phrase, "Rue the day," meaning you will regret it. The word *rue*, from the genus *Ruta*, means "to set free," and it was used in ancient times to treat poisonous bites. In this ritual, rue sets us free from poisons held in the heart. Also known as the herb of grace, rue helps us release the regrets that surround the heart and prevent the flow of love.

### THE RITUAL

You'll need a metal garbage pail, as old and rusty as you can find, as it represents old garbage that we have no need for. The women gather in a circle, and each woman writes down a regret or bitter feeling about love or a relationship with which she continues to struggle. The bride begins by reading hers and says forcefully, "I let this go," and tosses it into the pail. Each woman takes a turn reading her regret and letting it go. When everyone has had a chance, the group takes the pail outside and lights the papers inside it on fire. While it burns, the women chant together, "We let this go, we let this go." Following the burning ritual, the women share coffee with rue and honey cayenne popcorn.

The food for this ritual is influenced from a traditional Ethiopian method of adding the herb rue to coffee before drinking. The combination of both of these bitter plants, rue and coffee, means that we are drinking in and digesting (and ultimately eliminating) any bitterness and regrets, and this bitterness is balanced by the sticky, sweet honey-covered popcorn. We recognize and embrace the bitter elements that influenced our lives, just as we release them and celebrate the sweetness ahead that will "stick" with us. The popcorn is served in a big bowl and the women sit around digging into the bowl, licking their fingers, loudly and exaggeratedly, to signify that "we are in this together," supporting each other, hearts open to life and relationships that are sweet and spicy, sticky and messy.

### ↠ *Rue Coffee and Honey Cayenne Popcorn* ↞

**COFFEE:** Prepare coffee as you wish and give each woman a sprig of fresh rue to stir in her cup, or alternatively you can add some dried seeds or dried herb to the coffee while brewing.

**POPCORN:** In a saucepan add ¼ cup of butter and a cup of raw local honey. Mix them together and add ½ teaspoon of African bird pepper or cayenne. Pour over 4 to 6 cups of hot popcorn and let cool. Serve in a large bowl.

## WEDDING/COMMITMENT CEREMONY: MAKING GIFTS IN THE POTLATCH TRADITION

There are numerous rituals you can create for your wedding or commitment day, but the one I love the most is where the couple gives gifts of herbs or spices to their guests. When my husband and I decided to get married, we wanted to create rituals that combined elements from our various cultural and spiritual traditions that meant a lot to us.

### THE RITUAL

The potlatch is practiced by many North American native peoples, and the idea behind this gift giving is that the more you give away, the wealthier you are. (This is in contrast to concepts that say the more you collect, the wealthier you are.) The potlatch shows: "I am wealthy in friends and material possessions, and I want to share them." Thus, one gives gifts to guests when they are getting married or making a commitment.

We decided to make mango chutney with a range of delicious spices. We then bottled and labeled it and gave it, along with cotton dish towels, to our friends and families, so they would receive items both delicious and practical. We made the gift making a ritual between us in the weeks prior to the ceremony and then after our marriage ceremony, we had a potlatch where we all gathered together and gifted our guests one by one with a gift and a statement about what makes them special and also special to us. Then we feasted.

You can make any gift you wish. It might be a potpourri blend with a label, a special mix of herbal teas, a fermented food, or something like the chutney that is rich in spices and will last in the fridge for a while.

## MOTHER-SHOWERING RITUAL

In the Jewish tradition one celebrates a child—after its birth and not before—in a naming ceremony. Similarly, in many cultures, as in many communities in Mexico, a child is named only after she makes her personality known so that a name reflects the qualities she begins to show even in the first weeks of life.

After the child has made their entrance into the world beyond their mother's womb, gifts for the child come next. This mother-showering ritual is where women can offer their energy, love, and support to the mother before she embarks on what will be one of the most challenging and enduring experiences of her life. It is with this in mind that the ritual for showering the mother is imagined.

### THE RITUAL

This ritual is designed to create a talisman imbued with positive blessings for the expectant mother to carry with her throughout the remainder of her pregnancy, labor, and childbirth. It can also be held as a protective amulet, to be given to the child when born or on a special birthday later in her or his life. Begin by having each person who is going to attend the showering collect a meaningful herb or mineral to include in the talisman.

The herbs might include one or more of the following:

- A piece of angelica root, the "angel" herb, to invoke protection for mother and child

- Lotus (*Nelumbo nucifera*) leaf, petals, or seeds to represent one's ability to transcend suffering and hardship

- A sprig of rosemary to call forth wisdom and mental fortitude

- A pinch of vervain, known as the enchanter's herb, to protect well-being

- A yarrow bloom, named for the warrior Achilles, to bring vitality and courage

Mineral offerings may include rose quartz to represent unconditional love, tiger's eye for tenacity and willpower, black onyx to ward off negativity, or moonstone for connection to the lunar power and one's innate sensuality. Whatever herbs or minerals are selected, let them be imbued with loving intention.

Once all are gathered as a group for the showering, each person presents her gift, placing it in front of the mother as a sacred offering, along with a brief explanation of its meaning. Then the gift giver lights a candle and places it at the edge of the gift collection, and this begins a circle of light surrounding the gifts. As each person offers her own gift to the talisman, the circle of light will grow to encompass and surround the collection of gifts. After the last person has stepped forward, the entire group joins hands around the mother and the offerings, enveloping all in a protective circle. The expectant mother can next offer a hope for the life that is soon to be entering this world, after which she can blow out the candles to release the invocation into the universe alongside the rising smoke.

The offerings should then be gathered by someone in the group and placed in a pouch for the expectant mother to carry with her throughout the final stages of her pregnancy and eventually into the birth of her child. The candles from the ceremony can be kept and lit during the birth as a representation of the blessing each person offered in anticipation of this new life force.

Finally, a snack or meal may be shared with all.

## WELCOMING AN ANIMAL COMPANION TO OUR HOME

Not all of us will give birth to a child; we may birth and mother in many other ways. We welcome children in the neighborhood who need mothering, we teach or foster or adopt, and we also welcome animals into our lives as companions or for service or emotional support. This calls for a celebration and gathering as we engage family and friends to meet our new family member.

## THE RITUAL

Just as herbal medicines play an important role in our lives, so too do herbs help our animal friends stay healthy or regain health. It is important to know the specific needs of each species as what may be healthy for us, may be poison for our companions. What may be good for dogs, may not be good for cats. I have had the pleasure of living with both dogs and cats. This ritual focuses on welcoming a dog and creating an herbal medicine kit. If welcoming a cat or another animal, adjust the ritual to their needs.

In this ritual, we ask our friends and family to each bring a specific herbal remedy to help us build our first aid and herbal kit for our companion. Then we all sit in a circle on the floor and welcome the puppy or dog (or cat) by each person gently touching the dog one at a time and whispering sweet somethings into her ear and giving her a teeny treat while doing so. The role of touch is central to the socialization of humans, and dogs are no different. Practicing some touch techniques, while giving a treat such as massaging the ear flaps or the belly, gently stroking the paws, and massaging the gums, helps the dog feel safe and connected with new people. After everyone has had the opportunity to do this, cookies and tea are served while the group celebrates the new arrival by sharing each gift and explaining what it is good for and placing it in a herbal health basket. The following list provides some suggestions for herbal remedies that are good for dogs.

### REMEDIES FOR THE DOG HERBAL HEALTH BASKET

- Milk thistle for liver health
- Activated charcoal for accidental poisoning
- Calendula herbal paw salve
- Herbal flea collar
- Herbal shampoo
- Rescue Remedy
- Antianxiety, noise, and travel remedies including chamomile, valerian, and passionflower

## BIRTH AND LA CUARENTENA

When I first arrived in Mexico, *la cuarentena* was widely practiced. *La cuarentena* literally translates as "quarantine" and is the forty-day period when a woman rests after giving birth. She abstains from sex, eats lots of nourishing foods and herbs, and is cared for by her female friends and relatives who cook and clean and support almost all of her needs. Traditionally, women cover their heads and don't wash their hair because of the belief that one is vulnerable to various winds and drafts. La cuarentena is being practiced less frequently due to the demands of modern life. Even among rural women, la cuarentena is disappearing, and yet there is so much wisdom in providing women with unfettered time to bond with her newborn, while being relieved of all the pressures of caring for others. What a marvelous gift to give the new mother, to whatever degree possible, so that she is the focus of care and support.

**THE RITUAL**

Organize a group of friends and family members to review the needs of the new mother. They may include food preparation, cleaning with herbal products and aromatherapy, pitching in to serve as a nanny, a wet nurse, or lactation consultant, having someone sleep over to help soothe a crying baby, or arranging for laundry and house cleaning and food preparation. Provide a gift of an all-natural skin brush with instructions to dry brush skin daily toward the heart. This will keep the immune system strong and also speed the release of swelling fluids collected during pregnancy. Here is an adaptogenic recipe to prepare that provides nourishment to the blood and strength to the adrenal glands.

↠ *Postpartum Restoration* ↞

After giving birth, foods rich in minerals that support blood enrichment, along with the adaptogenic herbs, are especially helpful. The following recipe can be adapted for meat eaters or vegetarians. Lentils are rich in iron and minerals, and split peas are rich in potassium that will help move excess water retention. As an anti-inflammatory, rosemary helps heal delicate tissue and reduces pain after giving birth, and thyme helps maintain a good mood following the stress of childbirth. The adaptogenic herbs and mushrooms provide strength and restore energy.

↠ *Restorative Rosemary/Thyme Postpartum Soup* ↞

**SERVES 6**

6 cups bone, chicken, or
   vegetable broth
1 cup green lentils, rinsed

1 cup dried green peas, rinsed
1 cup sliced carrots
1 cup sliced celery

| | |
|---|---|
| 1 medium onion, sliced | 1 piece kombu |
| 2 cup chopped kale or chard | 5 fresh shiitake mushrooms, sliced |
| 3 cloves garlic, chopped | 1 teaspoon fresh ashwagandha root |

Place the lentils and peas in a slow cooker with the broth (as a general rule, use 3 cups of broth to each cup of dried lentils or peas). Add all the vegetables and roots and cook on low heat for 3 or more hours or until the lentils and peas are soft. You can also add a large sprig of rosemary and 1 teaspoon of fresh or dried thyme.

**OPTIONAL:** For the last hour of cooking add ¼ pound of sausage or chuck roast.

## SLEEPOVER WISHING WELL

This ritual is for four to six girls ranging from ages eight to thirteen.

Sleepovers are opportunities to release frustrations and share infatuations and build bonding skills among girls and young women. Creating the collective wishing well is a channel for identifying and sharing desires and releasing pent-up energy. It offers a ritual where each girl deepens her sense of self as she experiences the power and value of a collective of friends. While the host parent can facilitate, the mothers of the girls might enjoy gathering to support the initial phase of the ritual. This models female friendship and ritual.

### THE RITUAL

Plan this event during a full or new moon. Calendula—also known as English pot marigold—is the thematic flowering plant for a young girl's slumber party wishing well. Historically, the flowers have been used in devotional offerings to cast out negative energy and to cast love spells. Calendula's golden colors and aroma exude warmth, are associated with luck, and reinforce the ability to manifest one's hopes and dreams.

Gather a large batch of fresh calendula flowers and fill a large bowl with water. Have three additional bowls filled with sage, thyme, and marjoram. Have the girls sit in a circle, each taking a handful of flowers for themselves. Place the bowl of water in the middle of the circle and invite each girl to take turns putting their flowers in the bowl one at a time. Instruct them to say out loud a wish or desire with each addition to the bowl. When the wish is said out loud, in unison the girls should repeat the wish while placing a flower head in the water. Go around the circle twice so that each girl can share two wishes each. Once everyone has had a chance to add their flowers and wishes, they then take turns sealing the flower bowl ceremoniously by each placing a pinch or two of the herbs: sage for protection and the granting of wishes, thyme for the courage to pursue one's dreams, and marjoram for happiness.

Then place the bowl outside under the moon, or in the room where the girls sleep. In the morning, strain and bottle the essence into individual bottles so that each girl can take one home and remember her wishes, hopes, and dreams and those of her companions.

## COMING OF AGE

Spiritual rituals, like medical practices, reflect cultural values and evolve over time. Coming-of-age rituals are no different. I grew up in the conservative Jewish tradition in the 1950s in suburban Boston and was given a Bat Mitzvah, unlike my mother who was raised in a more orthodox tradition. Until the twentieth century, this ritual was reserved for boys coming of age. As women's rights and equality continue to be recognized, so too do the rituals that celebrate young girls and women. My Bat Mitzvah thus reflected its time and epoch. I loved learning the Torah and singing my part, but the ritual was considered de rigueur, and it was mostly about a party and family gathering. Yet I had no real sense of what was going on, and this may be in part because this ritual was also being performed in the context of "assimilation," or fitting in—so important to Jews of my parent's generation. In this sense, rituals often perform an essential function that continues cultural or spiritual traditions but does so in a way that obscures or hides their real meaning. We also see this in many cultures around the world where ceremonies (and their herbs) go underground in the face of being banned and then with their reemergence we are reminded of survival.

As a budding feminist at the age of thirteen, I was deeply attracted to the female bodhisattva Guan Yin. She embodies compassion and reduces the suffering of others. It was only as an adult that I discovered that the religion I was raised in, but did not adhere to, had a similar concept filled with meaning and purpose that I could embrace. It is called *tikkun olam*, the call to heal and transform the world through acts of kindness. This has informed my embrace of many of the world's cultures and ceremonies by which I explore my deepest purpose and meaning in life.

When my friend Jill's daughter had her Bat Mitzvah over thirty years after my own, times had changed and I was honored to be asked to facilitate a ritual of purpose and meaning that would add to a gathering of women after the Torah reading and party. All spiritual traditions have a similar concept and whether we are driven by a sense of spirituality or social justice, coming of age is about celebrating entry into adulthood, finding purpose and meaning, and absorbing the wisdom of elders while also now being ready to participate actively to reduce the suffering of others.

For this ritual, I felt there were two goals: to receive the wisdom of the elders and to listen to how they had chosen to create positive change in the world. This ritual can be conducted as an all-female coming-of-age ceremony as part of a more organized effort at a temple, church, mosque, or coven or outside of any religious or spiritual context. It can also be enacted at any age that reflects the moment in time to celebrate the young woman's transition into a new important stage of life that adds self-agency as she solidifies her identity.

## THE RITUAL

This ritual is designed to last about ninety minutes and is followed by a shared meal or dessert. Ask your daughter who she would like to have join in her ritual. You might provide a suggested list of up to eight women. Each invited woman will share and speak, so including only eight people keeps the time manageable. These participants should represent the many women who have been important to your daughter. They may include aunts and grandmothers, sisters, or teachers—mostly older women who have some wisdom to share with her. While younger female siblings may be invited, they are only observers.

Then ask your daughter to list favorite foods that she would like to share and include some favorite herbs with a blend of aromas. In advance of the ritual, gather together pots filled with herbs, such as lemon balm, oregano, basil, and lavender. You will need enough pots for each woman attending to have one.

Your daughter will write a special note of thanks to each participant in advance and pick out a pot of herbs for each one. She will research the meaning of the herb and its medicinal value. A handwritten note of just a few lines on beautiful notepaper provides a link for your modern young woman to rituals of the past. For example, lemon balm is known as the elixir of life and perhaps she wishes to give this to her aunt or a special auntie friend who has shown her what joie de vivre means. Or perhaps she knows a participant who loves to cook and would like to give her a pot of fresh basil, while sharing with her that basil enhances one's strength and is the sacred herb of Venus, the goddess of love. Whatever your daughter wishes to share, this represents her part in the ritual in which she gives to elders who have given to her.

Ask the invited women to wear very loose, comfortable clothing as a sign of being comfortable in one's own skin. (They may even decide to toss away their bras!) Let the guests know in advance what the ritual will entail so they may prepare. As the women gather, take off their shoes, and get seated comfortably, use a diffuser with your daughter's favorite essential oil, perhaps rose, lavender, or ylang ylang. Then serve her favorite herbal tea—it might be a chai or chamomile. Some of the women might also enjoy a botanical infused liqueur like damiana cognac (see "Crones' Ceremony" recipes on pages 248–49).

The ritual begins with the youngest woman guest. She will share a moment of her deepest wisdom; a phrase or an idea that is something your daughter can use her whole life. She will talk for a few minutes, telling a personal story from her own life and how this wisdom guided her and gave her strength. She will also share how she has made the world a better place, engaged in social justice, or helped others. She then gives the young woman a material gift, not one of financial value, but one that represents the wisdom she has shared that the young woman can keep as a reminder. Each woman goes around and speaks in the same way.

When the whole group is done, the young woman then speaks. She has on a table all of her handwritten cards and pots of herbs, and she stands and says something to each woman. Starting again with the youngest woman, she may respond to what the woman shared, thanking her, and also share why she chose this particular herb pot for her. She then continues around to the rest of the women and shares with each one. At the end of the ritual, the facilitator calls it completed and everyone stands and takes turns hugging each other. Then a meal or dessert can be shared.

## THE CYCLE OF CHANGE:
## RITUALS FOR MENARCHE AND MENSTRUATION

These rituals are intended to celebrate the meaning of menarche—the arrival of menstruation—as an encouraging and reassuring experience, enhanced by the support of older women who offer guidance and advice. The first menstruation can be an uneasy, confusing time for a young girl, especially if she has been exposed to popular culture or negative stories. As the body changes, hormones flow and unfamiliar emotions surge. A celebratory ritual of a girl's first menstruation can instill feelings of delight and honor for this sacred stepping-stone. If it can be scheduled during the full moon or the new moon you can explore the meaning of the moon in regulating women's cycles and the interrelationship between the flow of women's tides and the ocean's tides to build awareness about how lunar cycles affect the body and the Earth.

I also share ancient stories of lives of the different goddesses from various cultures to instill a sense of pride and ancestral connection. One story I especially love is about Hebe, the goddess of youth. Her mother was Hera, the goddess of women and queen of the heavens, and Hebe was born after her mother was impregnated by eating wild lettuce. Hebe served rich ambrosias, associated with sustaining the life force to the gods and goddesses. In the nineteenth century, water fountains were designed in her image, spurred by the female temperance movement to provide alternatives to alcohol and to represent drinking in moderation at a time of unchecked alcohol abuse and domestic violence against women. Hebe is also associated with the pomegranate, which can be a fun and deliciously messy fruit for the girls to eat during these rituals (its red juice symbolizing menstrual flow). Don't worry about "messiness."

## THE RITUAL: MAKING LAVENDER SACHETS

Lavender is a fragrant, hardy plant with relaxing properties. It is associated with love and fertility and is an excellent herb for a girl's menstrual rite of passage into womanhood. Invite a small group (four to six) of female family members and friends to your home. These women should be positive, self-assured, and serve as role models for your daughter's entry into womanhood. Women with diverse sexual orientations are particularly valuable as participants. Your daughter can also ask a few of her close friends to join.

Gather bundles of fresh lavender from the farmers market or harvest them from your backyard or a lavender farm. Provide scissors, muslin, and ribbons, or more simply, cotton bags with drawstrings. Provide a rolling pin or a mortar and pestle to grind down the lavender into a coarse powder. If you have lavender essential oil, mix a few drops into the powder. Have everyone fill their sachets with the mixture.

While making the sachets each woman takes a few minutes to share funny stories and their own positive experiences about what menarche was like for them and what their special tips are for embracing their flow and to offer words of reassurance and guidance to your child, making her feel especially loved and worshipped. This part is critical to instilling a sense of empowerment and pride in her menstrual cycle. At this stage, while one would not deny challenges, one should be discreet and not share horror stories either. The shared stories might also include a discussion about how each woman learned to set boundaries and stay safe and strengthened her capacity to say no, to anyone who asks for or demands access to her body and mind.

Once the sachets are finished, serve peppermint tea and cookies. At this time your child can ask any questions or lingering concerns about menarche, ovulation, or fertility, and women can take their turns providing answers. Above all this should be a time of laughter, trust, and caring.

Your daughter's sachet can be used as a stress reliever in times of overwhelming emotions. A larger sachet can also be made and warmed up in the oven or microwave for 2 minutes and used as an abdominal compress for menstrual cramps.

### THE RITUAL: MENARCHE CELEBRATION WITH A GROUP OF GIRLS

This ritual is designed to do with a group of girls around the same age over a period of weeks and months. It can be done a lunar month after making the lavender sachets (see page 243) or whenever you wish to gather a group of girls together. Because menarche begins at different times for girls, your daughter can call together a group of girls at any stage—those who are premenarche or those who are already menstruating. What is important is that they experience this together. This ritual is made up of a series of mini rituals where the girls learn how to do things for themselves (and each other) that will ease any discomfort they experience.

### THE RITUAL: GODDESS OF THE FLOW COLLAGE

Gather magazines with diverse colorful images along with art supplies like scissors, glitter, shells, pebbles, glue, tape, and so on.

The girls each imagine that they are the Goddess of the Flow—the universal energy that oversees the blood flow for all girls—and that this flow brings gifts of creativity and the power of friendship each month. Each girl then makes an art collage with images that symbolize her flow, the gifts she delivers, and images of lasting friendships and dreams fulfilled. Take about one hour or less to create this. Then have a snack of Goddess of the Moon Flow tea (recipe follows) and freshly made ginger cookies. During the snack each girl takes a turn and shares her flow collage and what it means to her.

---

→ *Goddess of the Moon Flow Tea* ←

**MAKES 4 CUPS**

Cinnamon, red raspberry leaf, and chamomile help the blood flow with ease.

Gently simmer 1 small cinnamon stick in 4 cups of water until the water is golden. Turn the heat off and add a teaspoon each of red raspberry leaf and chamomile flowers. Let sit for 15 minutes, then strain and serve.

---

## ↠ *Ginger Flow Cookies (Gluten Free)* ☜

Ginger softens menstrual cramps and warms the belly. The nutmeg, cinnamon, and cardamom also ease the flow. The molasses provides much-needed iron.

**MAKES 3 DOZEN COOKIES**

¼ cup whole cream

½ cup soft butter

¾ cup blackstrap molasses

1 egg

1 teaspoon vanilla

2 cups gluten-free flour mix (choose
    from combinations of buckwheat,
    rice, almond, potato, or tapioca flour)

½ cup diced crystallized ginger

1½ tablespoons baking powder

2 tablespoons ground ginger

1 teaspoon ground cinnamon

½ teaspoon ground nutmeg

½ teaspoon ground cardamom

¼ teaspoon sea salt

1 tablespoon plain yogurt

Preheat the oven to 375°F. To a large mixing bowl, add the cream, butter, and molasses and mix until combined. Add the egg and vanilla and beat well. In another bowl, mix together the flour, crystallized ginger, baking powder, ground ginger, cinnamon, nutmeg, cardamom, and sea salt. Add this to the butter and molasses mixture and mix well but don't overmix. Fold in the yogurt.

Prepare a cookie sheet with parchment paper. Roll the dough into small balls and place them on the prepared cookie sheet. Bake for 10 to 12 minutes. Remove from oven, let cool, and serve.

### RITUAL: BELLY STONE FOR EASING CRAMPS

The following ritual is about learning how to relieve any cramping or discomfort and includes making a fomentation and learning to rest in the mariposa pose.

If you are near a location where you can search for smooth oval or round river stones, then you can have the girls find their own stones as part of the ritual. Otherwise you can purchase basalt stones used for hot stone massage (online at a massage supply store in advance) and give the girls each three stones.

Add the stones to a slow cooker with enough water to cover them and heat on low or heat them in boiling water on the stove and then remove them with a slotted spoon. Whichever method is used, be careful not to get burned. Do not use a microwave to heat the stones, as it heats the stones unevenly and can be dangerous. You will use these stones with the following fomentation.

## ⇟ *Making a Fomentation* ⇐

A fomentation is the application of a warm, moist compress to a part of the body, often to ease pain and induce relaxation. Learning how to do this can be fun and informative for a group of girls, and the skill will last a lifetime.

To make a fomentation to reduce menstrual discomfort, start by combining ½ cup coarsely chopped fresh ginger, ½ cup cramp bark, and ½ cup American skullcap flowers, leaves, and stems in 4 cups of water. Simmer for 20 minutes and then turn off the heat. Strain the mixture and then dip a small wash cloth in it, wring it out and apply directly to the abdomen. Then cover the belly with a dry towel and place the hot stones on top. Rest and relax for 20 minutes while in the mariposa pose (instructions follow).

## ⇟ *Resting Mariposa Pose for Cramp Relief* ⇐

*Mariposa* means "butterfly" in Spanish. The butterfly represents metamorphosis and change from one cycle of nature to the next. Each month of our cycles reminds us of change and our link to the rhythms of nature. This position is designed to relieve cramping and discomfort during the flow. Rather than fight pain, this exercise asks us to say hello to the pain of cramps, to breath and relax without resisting and, instead, allow the pain to flow and then release. You can do this exercise after applying the fomentation and your belly is warm, or without the fomentation as time permits.

For the first part of this exercise, lie back on your bed with a pillow under your head and shoulders. Place the soles of your feet together, letting your legs fall wide open. If you need to support your legs, you can place some pillows underneath each of the knees. Feel for your pubic bone. This is a short, horizontal bone that is at the lowest part of your abdomen. Feel the tenderness in the bone. Use your thumbs to apply pressure against the bone and release the tenderness all along the bone.

Now, as you find the sensitive points, apply gentle pressure and breathe in to a count of 4, hold to a count of 4, release to a count of 4, and pause to a count of 4. Repeat this process for 10 minutes. Apply a little coconut oil on the abdomen and then a drop or 2 of lavender oil over that; gently rub the oils in a circular motion as you do this exercise.

## THE "WHAT'S NEXT" RITUAL

During the first dozen years I lived in the jungle, I lived outside, covered only by a thatched palm roof and some low walls that only gave an impression of a boundary. There was no electricity and thus no interference with my own natural energy fields, and this enhanced my telepathic experiences. I listened to the rhythm of ocean waves as they changed each lunar night, falling asleep to the moon and Venus in communion overhead. Thus began my practice of magic; of telepathy, intentionality, lucid dreaming, and receptivity. I lived where there was no phone service, and mail might arrive after a two- to three-week journey over land from the United States.

One night I dreamt that my grandfather Charlie had died, and when I awoke I just knew it was true. The next night I dreamt again about my grandfather but this time with more detail, and in the dream I was told that he had died of a heart attack. The third night I dreamt I was flying overhead in the temple in Boston during his funeral service, and I saw everyone in mourning. When I awoke I knew that he had come to me to say goodbye. Three weeks later the letter arrived sharing all of these details and dates. This was among the first of countless dreams I have had that relay the present or future from a distance, and this was how I began asking for deep information and guidance for next steps. I do this ritual when I want to tune in to "what's next," and you can do this also to strengthen your "dream muscle."

In our lives, we are often faced with what I call the "What's next?" We ask, "Do I take this path or that?" "Do I make this leap or hold back?" It might be a job or a relationship, or we might have finished a major phase of our lives: "Should I go to college?" "Do I travel or take that job offer?" "Do I have children now or wait?" Or, if the chickadees have flown the coop, "Now what?" Or we may have retired or simply be reexamining purpose and meaning in our lives. And always we ask the question: "What's next for me?" It is during these times that I conduct this three-night ritual.

### THE RITUAL

Gather twigs and branches and add them to a large basket to create a large nest to hold your hopes, dreams, and wishes for what's next. Place it next to your altar. Obtain a fresh peony and place it in a vase on your altar. The peony symbolizes compassion, which is central to reaching deeply into your future self.

Fill a pouch with about 2 ounces of zacatechichi (*Calea zacatechichi*) and place it under your pillow. Leave a little dried zacatechichi in a large shell or bowl to burn.

Write your question down on a piece of paper. Be very specific because the cosmic mind responds to specificity. Place the paper under the bowl holding the dried zacatechichi and then burn the zacatechichi.

Prepare a cup of valerian root tea and drink it 30 minutes before bed. This tea will enhance dreaming states. After you drink your tea, go to sleep on your right side. Lying on the right side deactivates the left brain and enhances right brain function. As you fall asleep ask your question specifically and repeatedly. When you wake in the night or morning, write down the dreams, images, or words that arise, but do not analyze them. Repeat this ritual for three nights in a row. On the fourth day read your writing, and you will very likely find the answer in the information gathered from your dreams.

## CRONES' CEREMONY

Gather together up to thirteen women who have reached menopause for this ritual.

A crone is a wise woman, a healer, an herbalist, and possibly a disagreeable old hag. In short, she has no more estrogen, the hormone of accommodation, and now that it's gone, so is the accommodation. This ritual celebrates the self, the wisdom acquired with age, and the spirit of "no one to please but myself." It also celebrates friendships, physical and cognitive flexibility, and core strength.

The herbal theme centers around the use of damiana and ginger. At least four weeks before the gathering date give each woman instructions to bring a food dish made with a selection of these hormonal herbs. One woman each can make the ginger massage oil, vanilla-infused honey, and the damiana-infused honey, and the hostess can make the damiana cognac (all recipes follow). The others can provide fruits like apples and pears, fresh and dried figs, and walnuts for dipping in the infused honeys and with their own special herbal gifts that celebrate wise women.

### → *Ginger Massage Oil* ←

Add 1 cup of freshly grated ginger (skin included) to 1 cup of coconut oil and simmer gently over low heat for 3 hours. Let cool slightly, strain through a fine strainer or cheesecloth, and bottle and label.

### → *Damiana Cognac* ←

**MAKES 4 CUPS**

Begin making this about 4 weeks in advance. Some people use vodka, but I prefer the natural sweetness of cognac, which goes well with the spicy feistiness of damiana. Plan for 2 to 3 ounces of beverage per woman attending, so adjust your ingredient amounts accordingly.

To a wide-mouth amber glass jar, add 5 ounces of damiana leaves to 1 quart of cognac or Armagnac. Cap tightly. Let it sit on a dark shelf for 4 weeks, shaking daily. At the end of the month, strain the leaves completely with a fine cheesecloth, making sure there is no residue. Rebottle the beverage in the original cognac bottle and label with the drink name and date.

## → *Damiana Tea* ←

**MAKES 1 SERVING**

Add 2 teaspoons of dried damiana leaves to 1 cup of boiled water, let sit for 15 minutes, strain, and sweeten with damiana-infused or vanilla-infused honey (recipes follow). Adjust this recipe based on how many women will be drinking the tea.

## → *Vanilla Infused Honey* ←

**MAKES 2 CUPS**

Cut 2 vanilla pods in half lengthwise and scrape out the seeds from inside the pods. Put the seeds and the pods in a clean glass pint jar and fill the jar to the top with a mild raw local honey. Cap tightly. Set the jar in a dark place and turn every day or so over a 2 to 4 week period. Remove the pods before use.

## → *Damiana Honey* ←

**MAKES 1 CUP**

Put ½ ounce of dried damiana leaves in a saucepan with 1 cup of honey and bring to a simmer. Remove from heat, strain the herb out when warm, and allow to cool. Cover and store in the dark.

## THE RITUAL

Begin by pouring the damiana beverage. (If any of the participants do not drink alcohol, make the damiana tea and damiana and vanilla honeys in advance and ensure that they feel comfortable participating in a ritual where women may drink. Or, if the majority of your participants do not drink, then choose the nonalcoholic damiana tea.)

Sit comfortably and as you drink, share sensuous, nourishing food chosen by each participant. Have each woman tell a story about her life. Share your earliest memory of who you thought you would be and bring it forward to the present, making the connections to who you have become and where you are going. For dessert, dip fruits and nuts in the leftover honey until the honey is gone, signifying a life well sated.

# RITUAL HONORING THE LOSS OF
# A HUMAN OR ANIMAL COMPANION

We can lose our human and animal companions at any moment, and it becomes one of the most profound experiences of our lives. I was fortunate to pass my adolescence with no losses of family or friends, but since I entered my twenties, they have been seemingly nonstop, with the loss of nearly thirty women friends over the years, most all to cancer. I have also mourned the loss of my parents and my three dogs. Each time I have learned something about loss and how painful and unwelcome it is, and how ritual can soothe the pain and bring me closer to my loved ones, both alive and dead.

Rosemary has long signified deep friendship and lasting memories. It is also the herb that will help to guide the loved one to their next place, support us through grief, and help us celebrate the life of our loved one.

## THE RITUAL

First, identify a place in your home where you will create an *ofrenda*, or an altar for your loved one, for a month-long period. Begin by gathering bunches of rosemary, either from the garden, from friends, or from the store. Tie these bunches together at the end and hang them upside down near the doorways of your home to dry.

Then gather items that represent the four elements of nature: fire, air, water, and earth. You may choose any object that has meaning for you; there is no right or wrong choice. For the fire element, a candle, incense, ashes, or hot spices work well. Air is associated with the colors blue, yellow, and white along with wood, so any wooden objects with these colors might be something to choose. The water element might be represented by a bowl of water or a photograph of your favorite body of water. For the earth element you might consider something that comes from the earth: dirt, a root, a gem, or something made from clay. Surround the altar with these objects so that it is embraced by the forces of nature. Engage family members and friends who want to participate. Young ones might make some art or items to add to the basket. Gather photographs from the earliest to the last days of your loved one.

As family and friends come to celebrate, they enter the home and remove their shoes. They then join in pairs, and each pair takes a bunch of rosemary. One person holds the rosemary while the other takes a light cotton string and wraps it several times around and along the length of the bunch so that the thick bunch of sprigs and branches becomes a tightly wound wand.

While the string is being wound, the pair looks each other in the eyes and says, "The circle of life goes round and round, the circle of life goes round and round. We celebrate the life of [Name]. The circle of life goes round and round."

When everyone is finished, they gather in a circle. One person lights their wand at the tip until the rosemary starts to smoke and then, holding the wand, they weave in and out of the circle, bathing each member in smoke. When they return to where they started, they hand the wand to their partner who does the same thing. Once that person has circled the entire group, the next person lights their wand and makes their trips around the circle. This continues until each person in the circle has had an opportunity to weave in and out holding their wand.

Following the circle, individuals might add small meaningful items to the ofrenda basket, and then everyone gathers around the table to eat the favorite foods of the loved one and share stories and photographs. As people depart, they may leave their wand at the altar and exchange it for another person's wand one month later to signify the enduring connections with each other and through the loved one who has journeyed on.

CAUTION: If this ceremony is done inside, good ventilation should be provided, and people with respiratory issues might want to sit this out at a distance.

### → Baked Pears and Rosemary ←

This pear recipe is sweet and tempered by a touch of rosemary as a reminder that this loved one's life brought much sweetness, but there is also sadness at their departure. The recipe is also fast and easy to prepare, signifying how quickly life changes.

Preheat the oven to 350°F and grease a cooking sheet. Slice three ripe Bartlett pears in half and take out the seeds and core, so there is a little gully in the middle of each. Fold a fresh rosemary sprig or two and tuck it into the center of each pear, along with a few raisins. Place the pears cut-side down on the prepared baking sheet and drizzle them with maple syrup. Bake for 45 minutes. Serve with a cup of Hot Coconut Kava (recipe follows).

## → Hot Coconut Kava ←

Kava is used traditionally in Hawaii and Polynesia to recognize notable moments in life, like loss. Kava helps us experience feelings of grief without numbing the feelings. Because kava can be mildly stimulating, I suggest not drinking this drink after 5:00 PM. If children participate in this ritual make them a special children's drink using the same recipe but without the kava.

**SERVES 6**

1 to 2 ounces kava root (¼ to ½ ounce ground powder kava root per person)

One 13.5-ounce can coconut cream or coconut milk

1 cup hemp milk

1 teaspoon ground cinnamon or half a cinnamon stick

Pinch of cardamom

1 tablespoon ghee or raw butter

2 drops vanilla or small piece of vanilla pod

10 drops stevia

Put all the ingredients except the ghee, vanilla, and stevia in a saucepan over medium heat. Simmer for 30 minutes. Remove from heat and strain out the kava root and cinnamon stick. Add the ghee, vanilla, and stevia. Froth to blend and serve hot.

# CONCLUSION

As a devotee of the goddess in all her forms, I was vistited early in my life by Guan Yin, the female bodhisattva of compassion. I had been a devotee for over a decade when one day, I was driving along a narrow country road seeking solace in nature from a very traumatic event. I passed a gas station and then a country store a few miles later.

Then suddenly I saw an orange and green flashing neon sign screaming "mattress store." I thought this was a strange sight in the middle of a quiet, two-lane country road, and I certainly didn't need a mattress, but I was drawn beyond my will to park and walk into the store. There, at the entrance, was the reason I had been beckoned. Standing before me was a three-foot ceramic Guan Yin smiling and greeting me with her open palm. I felt as though I had run into a long-lost friend. I then saw her bright orange pendant, which was a price tag, hanging from her neck, and as I inspected her closely I discovered that she had a huge crack where her head met her neck. It had been glued back together, and I laughed and thought, "Well, if Guan Yin can lose her head and get glued back together, then so can I!" I picked her up and carried her to my car, and she has traveled with me ever since, an ever-ready reminder of the power of compassion, synchronicity, and the need to always carry glue.

I make Guan Yin Tea before I sit in quiet contemplation. The preparation allows me to quiet my mind and body if I am feeling stressed or to take an hour alone in an otherwise busy life. I invite you to make yourself a cup of Guan Yin Tea every time you face what feels like an overwhelming challenge in your life or when you just want to connect with your inner, wise, guide. As you sip and breathe in and out, in and out, inhale your inherent strength of purpose, the strength befitting an Iron Goddess.

## ⇉ *Guan Yin Tea, a.k.a. Iron Goddess Oolong* ⇇

**MAKES 1 SERVING**

Guan Yin tea is a highly prized variety of oolong that brings many healing properties. It is a mildly fermented tea, rich in antioxidants, low in caffeine, and a natural immune booster. There are many Buddhist stories about how Guan Yin tea evolved as a beverage in China. Traditionally, it is hand rolled into small, tight balls of black leaves, which some suggest are like heavy little iron balls, hence its name Iron Goddess tea or *tieguanyin*.

To make this fragrant tea, add 2 teaspoons of tea in an infuser in a glass tea mug. Boil 1 cup of water and infuse the tea for 3 to 5 minutes. Strain, sip, and enjoy.

As you continue to explore the healing role of herbal medicines in your life and experiment with the ideas, methods, and remedies that I recommend in this book, take some time to reflect on your deep capacity to heal yourself, your friends, and your family, and to enjoy the journey into the world of plant medicines, one that is meant to last a lifetime.

# → RESOURCES ←

## CONTACTING DR. LESLIE KORN

Readers of this book will find several additional resources of interest, including my clinical website (drlesliekorn.com), where I write a blog, post recipes, and have information about consultations. I also direct research at the Center for Traditional Medicine (cwis.org), where you will find resources about indigenous peoples, medicine, and online courses.

## BEFORE PURCHASING HERBAL MEDICINES

I have an account at Fullscript where I offer a discount for purchase of all herbal products. Proceeds of all sales support my nonprofit program, Nutrients for Natives, which brings herbal medicine to native peoples with diabetes. Sign up here: fullscript.com/practitioners/dr-leslie-korn.

## HERBAL MEDICINE PURVEYORS OF DRIED HERBS, EXTRACTS, AND SYRUPS

**Banyan Botanicals**

www.banyanbotanicals.com

Manufacturer and purveyor of Ayurvedic botanical products and accessories, including ashwagandha bala massage oil. They also maintain a blog for an Ayurvedic lifestyle.

**Biotics Research NW**

www.bioticsnw.com

A source of gastrazyme, valerian hops, and passionflower (V. H. P.), along with oregano oil and other herbs and high-quality nutrients.

**Gaia Herbs**

www.gaiaherbs.com

One of my favorite growers and retailers of proprietary herbal formulas in the form of capsules and extracts.

**Herb Pharm**

www.herb-pharm.com

I routinely use their tinctures, glycerites, capsules, and other prepared herbal
  medicine. They provide both simplers and their own proprietary formulas.

**Kalustyan's**

foodsofnations.com

An online and brick-and-mortar specialty food store in Curry Hill, Manhattan,
  offering a large array of foreign spices, medicinal teas, bulk herbs, and other global
  foods.

**Mountain Rose Herbs**

www.mountainroseherbs.com

An online botanical retailer offering a vast array of herbal products from bulk herbs to
  smoking blends, DIY products, and cosmetics. It's a one-stop shop for all your needs
  in herbal products.

**Organic India**

us.organicindia.com

Purveyor of teas, herbal extracts, and tulsi infusions, all sustainably sourced from
  wildcrafters and family farms in India.

**Pacific Botanical**

www.pacificbotanicals.com

Wholesale supplier and grower of fresh and dried herbs and spices, powders, and bulk
  seeds based in Applegate Valley, Oregon.

**Starwest Botanicals**

www.starwest-botanicals.com

Supplier of bulk herbs, herbal products, and accessories. They offer wholesale pricing
  for those interested in reselling.

**Urban Moonshine**

www.urbanmoonshine.com

Certified organic herbal extract purveyor specializing in herbal bitters and tonics.

**Wise Woman Herbals**

www.wisewomanherbals.com

Supplier of a variety of botanical supplements that employ ingredients sourced mostly
  from local farms in the Pacific Northwest.

## CANNABIDIOL (CBD) PRODUCT SUPPLIERS

### Citizen CBD

citizencbd.com

Founded by a veteran, Citizen CBD began as a form of medicinal support for people returning from combat. The company uses foreign imported hemp to make e-liquids, capsules, tinctures, and other consumables. Their gel capsules are considered the strongest on the market.

### Endobotanical LLC

Endoca.com

High-quality CBD medicines. I have arranged for a discount for the readers of this book: Use code Korn15

### Extract Labs

www.extractlabs.com

Based in Boulder, Colorado, and founded by a combat veteran, this lab offers a full-spectrum of CBD products. Lab analysis of each of their products is also provided.

### Populum

populum.com

Offering oils, rubs, and pet products using hemp grown on a farm in Colorado. Lab results of cannabinoid content (along with other compounds) are posted on their website.

### Sagely Naturals

https://www.sagelynaturals.com/

Offers two lines of CBD products: one addresses pain and inflammation and the other addresses stress and anxiety. Consumables and topicals available.

### USA Hemp

www.usahemp.com

High-quality CBD products for health. I have arranged for a discount for the readers of this book: Use code usak15.

## FUNGI PURVEYORS

**Fungi Perfecti**

www.fungi.com

Certified organic company specializing in gourmet and mushroom-related products. Founded by mycologist Paul Stamets, Fungi Perfecti grows, maintains, and harvests fungi for a line of formulary supplements.

**Gourmet Mushrooms**

www.gmushrooms.com

Online supplier of gourmet mushrooms, mushroom products, and mushroom-growing kits.

**Nammex Organic Mushroom Extracts**

www.nammex.com

Organic mushroom extract ingredient wholesale supplier.

**Real Mushrooms**

www.realmushrooms.com

Retail supplier of organic mushroom capsules and extract powders.


## HERBAL RESOURCES FOR TRANSGENDER, GENDERQUEER, AND NONBINARY PERSONS

**Competent Care for Transgender, GenderQueer, and Non-Binary Folks**

sites.google.com/vtherbcenter.org/transhealth/home

A compilation of resources for herbal practitioners curated by clinical herbalists Vilde Chaya Fenster-Ehrlich and Larken Bunce.

**Herbs for Trans*Gender Folx**

www.sfherbalist.com/articles

From herbalist Kara Sigler, a series of articles and presentations on competent herbal care.

**Holistic Health for Transgender and Gender Variant Folks**

www.ohlonecenter.org/wp-content/uploads/2017/06/Midnight_D_Transgender _Care.pdf

A paper on herbal approaches for trans and gender variant bodies written by Dori Midnight.

## HANDCRAFTED/WILDCRAFTED SMALL BATCH HERBS

### Avena Botanicals

www.avenabotanicals.com

Maine-based retailer offering handcrafted herbal remedies that are sourced from gardens and farms all over Maine.

### Blue Ridge Aromatics

blueridgearomatics.com

Based in Asheville, North Carolina, and specializing in craft essential oils. They hand distill essential oils and hydrosols on-site and source their plants from their own forest farm.

### Harding's Wild Mountain Herbs

www.hardingsginsengfarm.com

Growers and retailers of wild simulated ginseng and goldenseal located in the Appalachian Mountains in northwestern Maryland. They sell capsules, powders, berry concentrates, and ginseng seeds and raw roots.

### Ironbound Island Seaweed

www.ironboundisland.com

Purveyors of sustainably harvested wild seaweed from eastern Maine. They offer wild North Atlantic dulse, kelp, kombu, wakame, and nori.

### Organic Alcohol Co.

organicalcohol.com

Oregon-based organic distillery and online retailer of premium spirits for crafting botanical extracts.

### Pacific Botanicals

www.pacificbotanicals.com/store

Wholesale supplier and grower of fresh and dried herbs and spices, powders, and bulk seed based in Applegate Valley, Oregon.

### Pinenut.com

www.pinenut.com

Online retailer of American pinon pine nuts and other wild-growing crops. They are also a certified-organic wild native nursery in Missouri where all their products are harvested and cultivated sustainably.

**Sonoma County Herb Exchange**

www.sonomaherbs.org/herb-exchange

Co-op of twenty-five local farmers and growers in Northern California selling their
herbs at weekly markets in Sonoma County.

**Steadfast Herbs**

www.steadfastherbs.com

A quarterly shipment of five essential handmade herbal remedies in tune with
seasons. Made with herbs grown on a farm in Pescadero, California.

**Strictly Medicinal Seeds**

strictlymedicinalseeds.com

Online purveyor of organic medicinal seeds and seedlings.

**Tooth of the Lion**

toothofthelion.com

Shares available for three, six, or nine months and include boxes of seasonal medicines
created from their farm in Orwigsburg, Pennsylvania.

**White Pine Community Farm**

www.whitepinecommunityfarm.com

Based in Wingdale, New York. Offers a sliding-scale debit share, which includes a
10 percent discount off regular prices and exclusive access to certain herbs. Pick up
at farmers markets across New York; delivery options also available.

**Wild and Wise Herbal CSA**

www.wildandwisecsa.com

Based in Petrolia, California. Offers monthly CSA packages to shareholders each year.
They offer shares on a sliding scale.

## SPIRIT PLANT PURVEYORS

**Multidisciplinary Association for Psychedelic Studies (MAPS)**

maps.org

Founded in 1986, MAPS is a nonprofit research and educational organization that
develops medical, legal, and cultural contexts for people to benefit from the careful
use of psychedelics and marijuana.

**People of Color Psychedelic Coalition**

www.zoehelene.com/ifetayo-harvey

Ifetayo Harvey founded this group to address the marginalization of people of color
and psychedelics.

**Psychedelic Feminism**

www.zoehelene.com

Most well-known for popularizing the term and subgenre, *psychedelic feminism*, Zoe
Helene is also the founder of Cosmic Sister, an educational advocacy group that
connects women in mutually supportive ways, while promoting several other
interconnected advocacy groups (focused around sacred plants, indigenous rights,
cultural preservation, and sustainability).

**Psychēplants**

www.psycheplants.org

An information hub and e-health platform about psychoactive plants, from the
International Center for Ethnobotanical Education and Service.


## IBOGAINE CLINICS

*Please note that inclusion here does not warrant a recommendation
but rather a resource to explore with care.*


**Awakening in the Dream House**

San Miguel de Allende, Guanajuato

www.awakeninginthedream.com/index.html

**Clear Sky Recovery**

Cancun, Quintana Roo

clearskyibogaine.com

**Crossroads Research Initiative**

Bahamas

crossroadsibogaine.com

**Ibogaine Clinic**

Solidaridad, Quintana Roo

ibogaineclinic.com

## MEDIA AND CONFERENCES

### BotanicalMedicine.org

www.botanicalmedicine.org

A resource for conferences, webinars, audio recordings, and books that center on herbal medicine.

### The Herbal Highway

kpfa.org/program/the-herbal-highway

Hosted and produced by Karyn Sanders and Sarah Holmes, the podcast delves into herbal medicine and alternative healing practices. Episodes air on Thursdays at 1:00 PM Pacific time.

## INTERNSHIPS/APPRENTICESHIPS

### Alquimia Centre of Healing Arts

alquimiahealingarts.com

Based in the Amazon of Ecuador, the center offers an internship in herbal medicine and shamanism through the lens of ancestral wisdom and ethnobotany.

### American Botanical Council Internship

abc.herbalgram.org

Offers an internship program in Austin, Texas, in pharmacy, diet, botany, horticulture, journalism, and marketing.

### Cedar Mountain Herb School

www.cedarmountainherbs.com

Based in Seattle, Washington. Offers apprenticeships and community workshops with a focus on herbs of the Pacific Northwest.

### Eclectic Institute

www.eclecticherb.com

This institute offers an eight-week Budding Herbalist Internship Program in Sandy, Oregon. Traditional Western health practices are the main focus of the program, which includes classes and plant hikes.

### Heartstone Center for Earth Essentials

www.heart-stone.com

Based in Ithaca, New York. Offers on-site education in herbalism, an herbal apprenticeship program, and workshops.

### Herbaculture Internship Program at Herb Pharm

www.herb-pharm.com/connect/internship

Located in the Siskiyou Mountains in Oregon, the Herbaculture Internship is offered
in three sessions and includes work on Herb Pharm's botanical education garden
and training classes on plant identification, responsible wildcrafting, plant
communication, and more.

### Misty Meadows Herbal Center

www.mistymeadows.org/herbal-apprenticeship

Based in Lee, New Hampshire. Offers an eight-month program for beginners in herbal
healing that covers native plant identification and traditional and plant-spirit
medicines.

### Northeast School of Botanical Medicine

7song.com

Led by 7Song. Offers a Community Herbalism Intensive program, a Weekend
Herbalism program, and traditional apprenticeships in Ithaca, New York.

### Sawmill Herb Farm

www.sawmillherbfarm.com/internship

This small herb farm in western Massachusetts hires interns during the growing
season to help with all aspects of farming for medicinal and culinary herbs.

### Wildwood Institute

www.wildwoodinstitute.com

Based in Verona, Wisconsin. Offers one-, two-, and three-year apprenticeship
programs and plant walks.


## CONTINUING EDUCATION/ON-SITE TRAINING/WORKSHOPS

### Abor Vitae School of Traditional Herbalism

arborvitaeny.com

Based in New York City. Offers on-site training for practicing herbalists, including
certification programs and community classes with visiting master herbalists.

### Ann Arbor School of Massage, Herbal and Natural Medicine

www.naturopathicschoolofannarbor.net

Based in Ann Arbor, Michigan. Offers on-site naturopath diploma and massage
therapy diploma programs approved by the state of Michigan.

**The Ayurvedic Institute**

www.ayurveda.com

Based in Albuquerque, New Mexico. Offers on-site teachings of the Ayurvedic healing
tradition with its principal teacher, Dr. Vasant Lad, who is also the director of the
institute.

**Bastyr University**

bastyr.edu

Campuses in Washington and California. Offers degree programs in a number of
natural health modalities, including a bachelor's degree in herbal sciences.

**Blue Ridge School of Herbal Medicine**

www.blueridgeschool.org

Based in Ashville, North Carolina. Offers various on-site programs catered to varying
levels of experience in the art of herbalism.

**Botanologos School of Herbal Studies**

wildhealingherbs.com

Based in the southern Appalachian Mountains of Georgia. Offers an on-site
certification program in the foundations of herbalism as well as seminars and
workshops with a strong focus on the Appalachian flora.

**Cedar Mountain Herb School** (*See* "Internships/Apprenticeships")

**Chestnut School of Herbal Medicine**

chestnutherbs.com

Offering online courses and an herbal immersion program that explores all aspects of
herbal medicine, from growing your own herbal garden to medicine making and
creating a sustainable living from herbal medicine.

**Colorado School of Clinical Herbalism**

clinicalherbalism.com

Based in Boulder, Colorado. Offers on-site certification programs in medical herbalism
and clinical nutrition for varying levels of expertise.

**David Winston's School for Herbal Studies**

www.herbalstudies.net

Based in Washington, New Jersey. Offers an on-site and online certification program
in herbalist training.

**East West School of Planetary Herbology**

planetherbs.com

Based in Santa Cruz County, California. Offers on-site and offsite certification
    programs for clinical herbalism.

**The Eclectic School of Herbal Medicine**

eclecticschoolofherbalmedicine.com

Based in Lowgap, North Carolina. Offers online certification programs and on-site
    intensive programs in clinical herbalism.

**Foundations of Herbalism**

www.foundationsofherbalism.com

A correspondence herbalist training program led by Christopher Hobbs, with a focus
    on traditional Chinese and Western herbalism.

**Franklin Institute of Wellness**

franklininstituteofwellness.com

Based in Franklin, Tennessee. Offers on-site and online training in herbal medicine
    and aromatherapy. They have diplomas and certificate programs based on
    research-based courses.

**Genesis School of Natural Health**

genesisschoolofnaturalhealth.org

An online school offering diplomas for master herbalist, natural health consultant,
    holistic health professional, and traditional doctor of naturopathy.

**Grassroots Herbalism**

grassrootsherbalism.com

Offering online courses in medicine making and a twelve-week online course in
    herbal medicine. Grassroots also hosts a collective that is mentored by the school's
    founder, Don Ollsin, and webinars focused on herbalism, sustainability, and
    environmental education.

**Heart of Herbs Herbal School**

www.heartofherbs.com

Online certification programs for certified herbalist, master herbalist, certified
    aromatherapist, and clinical aromatherapist, as well as herbal skin care for
    business and flower essence certification.

**Heartstone Center for Earth Essentials** (*See* "Internships/Apprenticeships")

**Herbal Wisdom Institute**
www.herbalwisdominstitute.com
Based in Prescott Valley, Arizona. Offers a 300-hour Western herbalist certification
course, workshops, and plant walks.

**Maryland University of Integrative Health**
www.muih.edu
Based in Maryland with online learning options available. Offers continuing education
as well as master's- and doctoral-level training.

**New Eden School of Natural Health and Herbal Studies**
www.newedenschoolofnaturalhealth.org
A distance learning school with a variety of diplomas in health studies. They offer
certified herbalist, master herbalist, and medical herbalist programs, and a
certified herbal consultant diploma.

**Northeast School of Botanical Medicine** (*See* "Internships/Apprenticeships")

**Ohlone Herbal Center**
www.ohlonecenter.org
Based in Berkeley, California. Offers individual courses in Western herbal medicine
and a certification program for practicing clinical Western herbalism.

**Pacific Rim College**
www.pacificrimcollege.com
Based in Victoria, British Columbia. Offers both on-campus and online learning
options in a number of different holistic medicine modalities.

**The Science and Art of Herbalism**
scienceandartofherbalism.com
A distance learning course from Rosemary Gladstar.

**Southwest School of Botanical Medicine**
www.swsbm.com/HOMEPAGE/HomePage.html
Michael Moore's collected and digitized compendium of resources, including his own
teachings and experience in the field of medicinal plants.

**Traditions School of Herbal Studies**

www.traditionsherbschool.com

Based in St. Petersburg, Florida. Offers clinical training in Eastern and Western
medicine.

**Vermont Center for Integrative Herbalism**

vtherbcenter.org

Based in Montpelier, Vermont. Offers on-site clinical training in herbalism with
hands-on experience in a community clinic as well as workshops and short courses.

**Wildflower School of Botanical Medicine**

wildflowerherbschool.com

Based in Austin, Texas. Offers on-site herbal programs in introductory home and
family herbcraft, intermediate community herbcraft, and advanced clinical
herbcraft.

**Wildwood Institute** (*See* "Internships/Apprenticeships")

**Wintergreen Botanicals**

wintergreenbotanicals.com

Based in Bear Brook State Park in New Hampshire. Offers an on-site and online
Herbalist Intensive Training Program with certificate.


## HERBAL NUTRIENT DATABASES FOR POTENTIAL INTERACTIONS

**American Botanical Council**

abc.herbalgram.org

This nonprofit offers drug-herbal interactions for most commonly used therapies.
Just type the herbal supplement in the search and common interactions and
contraindications should come up.

**Express Scripts**

www.Drugdigest.org

A searchable database that covers 11,500 potential interactions, including drugs and
herbs.

**Herbal/Medical Contraindications**

www.swsbm.com/ManualsMM/HerbMedContra1.pdf

This document by Michael Moore outlines complications with specific herbs based
on their potentially harmful effects on different systems. Particularly useful is the
pregnancy section that outlines potentially harmful herbs for pregnant women.

**Integrative Therapeutics**

www.integrativepro.com/Resources/Drug-Nutrient-Interaction-Checker

This manufacturer of supplements provides a drug-interaction checker that offers
information on documented and theoretical interactions between drugs and
nutrients or herbs.

**RXList**

www.rxlist.com/supplements/article.htm

Supplement monographs available, which include potential safety concerns and
interactions with pharmaceuticals. Downloadable PDFs available outlining
herb-drug and nutrient-drug interactions. Monographs of the most commonly
encountered therapeutic agents and their potential interactions with
pharmaceuticals in easy-to-understand language.

## HERBAL ASSOCIATIONS

**American Botanical Council**

abc.herbalgram.org/site/PageServer?pagename=Herbal_Library

A research and education organization dedicated to providing accurate and reliable
information for consumers, health care practitioners, researchers, educators,
industry, and the media. They publish peer-reviewed articles, books, monographs,
and continuing education materials and maintain a database of all things related to
plant medicine.

**American Herbal Pharmacopoeia**

www.herbal-ahp.org

A nonprofit that publishes informative monographs on botanicals. Monographs
include plant chemistry, handling and processing, purity standards, side effects,
and drug interactions, among other information.

**American Herbal Products Association**

www.ahpa.org/Home.aspx

This is the trade association and voice of the herbal products industry. It consists
of businesses involved with manufacturing, processing, growing, and marketing
herbs and herbal products. Their mission is to promote responsible practices by
businesses and to keep consumers informed.

**American Herbalists Guild**

www.americanherbalistsguild.com

An association of herbalists established in 1989 that provides online resources in education, research, mentorship, and schools. The *Journal of the American Herbalists Guild* is the first peer-reviewed herbal medicine journal to contain articles in clinical herbalism and biomedicine.

**The Canadian Herbalist's Association of British Columbia**

www.chaofbc.ca

An organization of herbal practitioners and enthusiasts providing leadership and resources for herbal practitioners in Canada.

**The Herb Society of America**

www.herbsociety.org

An organization that champions the use of herbs as essential additions to our lives. They provide print and digital resources in herbal history and lore, growing tips, and medicinal uses of herbs.

**United Plant Savers**

www.unitedplantsavers.org

An organization dedicated to the conservation of threatened medicinal plants in the United States and Canada.

### HERBAL DATABASES

**Andean Botanical Information System**

www.sacha.org

A website dedicated to documenting relevant information regarding flowering plants of Andean South America.

**Dr. Duke's Phytochemical and Ethnobotanical Databases**

phytochem.nal.usda.gov/phytochem/search

A database of plants and data relevant to their chemistry, bioactivity, and ethnobotany.

**The Herbarium**

herbarium.theherbalacademy.com

From the Herbal Academy, an online database of herbal resources, including herbal monographs, articles, and educational tools.

**HerbMed**

www.herbmed.org

An herbal database that provides hyperlinks to scientific data related to the use of herbs as medicine.

**Holistic Online Herbal Directory**

www.holisticonline.com/Herbal-Med/Hol_Herb_Directory_Index.htm

An online database archiving medicinal herbs and relevant information. Includes proper dosages, safety information, uses, active compounds, and parts used.

**Medical Herbalism**

medherb.com/articles.htm

A website containing links and references to articles regarding the science, history, and art of medical herbalism.

**National Agricultural Library**

agricola.nal.usda.gov

One of four national libraries of the United States that contains a large collection of literature on agriculture and its related science. Its online database provides citations to agricultural literature.

**Native American Ethnobotany Database**

naeb.brit.org

A database containing plants and their ethnobotanical and medicinal uses by indigenous Americans.

**Plants for a Future**

www.pfaf.org/user/Default.aspx

A database of approximately 7,000 plants that provides ethnobotanical uses, habitats, physical characteristics, cultivation details, weed potentials, and other relevant scientific and horticultural facts.

**PubMed**

www.ncbi.nlm.nih.gov/pubmed

A database of references and abstracts on life sciences and biomedical topics.

**Raintree Tropical Plant Database**

www.rain-tree.com/plants.htm#.WoJ0tZM-eRs

A database of medicinal plants found in the Amazon, including their uses, chemical analysis, biological activities, and relevant clinical research. The website is run by Leslie Taylor and documents her own experience in the field.

**USDA PLANTS Database**

plants.usda.gov/java

Complete botanical information on plants growing in the United States. This includes
range maps, pictures, and endangered status.

## SCIENTIFIC JOURNALS

*The following journals contain peer-reviewed, up-to-date scientific research articles in their corresponding fields.*

**American Journal of Botany**

www.amjbot.org

**Fitoterapia**

www.journals.elsevier.com/fitoterapia

**International Journal of Herbal Medicine**

www.florajournal.com

**Journal of Alternative and Complementary Medicine**

online.liebertpub.com/toc/acm/24/1

**Journal of Ethnopharmacology**

www.sciencedirect.com/journal/journal-of-ethnopharmacology

**Journal of Herbal Medicine**

www.journals.elsevier.com/journal-of-herbal-medicine

**Journal of Medicinal Food**

online.liebertpub.com/loi/JMF

**Journal of Natural Products**

pubs.acs.org/journal/jnprdf

**Pharmaceutical Biology**

www.tandfonline.com/loi/iphb20

**Phytochemical Analysis**

onlinelibrary.wiley.com/journal/10.1002/(ISSN)1099-1565

**Phytochemistry**

www.journals.elsevier.com/phytochemistry/

*Phytomedicine*

www.journals.elsevier.com/phytomedicine/

*Phytotherapy Research*

onlinelibrary.wiley.com/journal/10.1002/(ISSN)1099-1573

*Planta Medica*

www.thieme.com/books-main/biochemistry/product/3494-planta-medica


## MAGAZINES, ONLINE REFERENCES, AND BLOGS

### The American Herbalists Guild

www.americanherbalistsguild.com

An association of herbal practitioners offering support and resources to the herbal
community. In 1989, the guild issued the first peer-reviewed clinical botanical
medicine journal called the *Journal of the American Herbalists Guild*. It continues
to be published biannually.

### *The Essential Herbal Magazine*

essentialherbal.com

A print magazine written by herbalists dedicated to herbal enthusiasts and herbal
businesses.

### Henriette's Herbal Homepage

www.henriettes-herb.com

Herbal medicine site run by Henriette Kress. Containing thousands of digitized
documents of classic manuscripts, herbal forum archives, botanical keys, and
relevant information regarding plant medicine.

### *The Herb Quarterly*

www.herbquarterly.com

The oldest herbal magazine providing plant-based recipes, resources on maintaining
medicinal gardens, up-to-date research in medicinal applications, and the history
and lore of herbs.

### *A Modern Herbal*

www.botanical.com

Digitized online copy of Mrs. M. Grieve's *A Modern Herbal*, published in 1931.
Contains scientific, anecdotal, and historical information on more than 800
varieties of plants and herbs.

**Natural Medicine Journal**

www.naturalmedicinejournal.com

An electronic journal and website dedicated to integrative health practitioners, students, faculty, and enthusiasts interested in natural medicine.

*Plants Are Magic Magazine*

rebeccadesnos.com/plants-are-magic-magazine

From botanical dyer Rebecca Desnos, a magazine that explores the relationship between people and plants through craft, herbalism, gardening, and storytelling.

**Traditional Medicinal's** *Plant Power Journal*

www.traditionalmedicinals.com/articles

Blog run by Traditional Medicinal's tea company that contains articles on herbalism.

# → INDEX OF HERBS ←
# IDENTIFIED IN THIS BOOK

# ⇉ INDEX ⇇

bile, function of, 143
biological cycles, 40–41
biomedicine, 1–2
bipolar disorder, 154, 205
bitter herbs, 7, 56, 70, 78, 80, 89, 92, 103,
　143–44
　for autoimmune disorders, 166
　for detoxification, 42
　in rituals, 234
　spices as, 116
　for stomachaches, 39
black currant seed oil, 147, 172, 174
black pepper, 140
　for brain health, 216–17
　essential oil, 140
　in spice blends, 120–21, 128–29
　turmeric and, 100, 147, 167
bladder, 34, 69, 88, 175–76. *See also*
　interstitial cystitis; urinary tract
　infections (UTIs)
blood pressure, 41
　foods for lowering, 209–10
　herbs for, 10, 40, 59, 79, 80, 82, 90, 92,
　95, 97
　low, 59, 128
　raising, 139
　sleep and, 153
　spice for, 122
blood sugar regulation, 10, 152, 226
　body conditioning and, 218
　herbs for, 66, 70, 73, 74, 75, 85, 89, 92
　osteoarthritis and, 188
　spices for, 110, 119, 126, 129
　stages of imbalance, 150–51
　*See also* diabetes
blueberries, 58, 117, 123, 212, 214, 216–17
body conditioning, 218–19
boils, 55, 74, 189
bone broth, 60–61, 148, 161–62, 188, 196,
　199, 238–39
bone health, 74, 186, 187–89, 215. *See
　also* osteoporosis
brain glandular powder, 216–17
brain health, 1, 59, 91, 96–97, 111, 135. *See*

*also* cognitive function
brandy and cognac, 19, 248–49. *See also*
　Armagnac
brassica vegetables, 45, 159, 208
breast cancer, 3, 67, 183
breastfeeding, 3, 9, 65–66, 89, 109, 183,
　184–85. *See also* galactagogues;
　lactation
breast health, 183–85
broccoli, 45, 46, 159, 214
bronchitis
　Anise Chest Rub and Anise Liqueur,
　109
　antispasmodics for, 34
　in children, 197–98
　in Chinese Medicine, 77
　herbs for, 59, 71, 75, 81, 84, 86, 87, 96
　Oxymel for Respiratory Health, 27
　spices for, 113, 124, 128, 129–30
brown sugar, 107–8
bruising
　herbs for, 23, 30, 39, 54, 57, 68, 71, 87,
　102
　in perimenopause, 185
　post-surgery, 195
　spices for, 105
burns, 36, 53, 57, 61, 64, 95, 102
butter, 115–16, 119–20, 245, 252. *See also*
　ghee

## C

cabbage juice, 37, 146
calcium supplementation, 188
cancer, 3, 155, 192
　fungi for, 75
　herbs for, 57, 66, 99
　pain from, 43
　seaweed for, 95
　soy and, 98
　spices for, 112–13, 125, 127
　spirit plants for, 135
　*See also* breast cancer; cervical cancer
cannabidiol (CBD), 33, 133–35, 160, 170,
　175, 178, 179, 225

# ➤ ABOUT THE AUTHOR ⬅

Leslie Korn, PhD, MPH, is a clinician specializing in mental health nutrition and integrative medicine for the treatment of chronic physical and mental illness. In 1975, she founded the Center for Traditional Medicine, a nonprofit public health clinic in rural indigenous Mexico that she has directed for over forty years. She served as a Fulbright Scholar on traditional medicine, a Clinical Fellow at Harvard Medical School, and a National Institutes of Health–funded research scientist in mind/body medicine. She is also the director of research at the Center for World Indigenous Studies. Author of nine books, Dr. Korn has a private practice and teaches and mentors internationally for mental health professionals and tribal communities. Her website is drlesliekorn.com.